wear this, toss that!

Hundreds of fashion and beauty swaps that save your looks, save your budget & save you time

AMY E. GOODMAN

A Stonesong Press Book

ATRIA BOOKS

New York   London   Toronto   Sydney

This book includes the author's opinions based on her research and experience, which reflect her independent judgment, formed without payment or expectation of payment from such companies. The author believes that information in this book is accurate as of the date of its first printing.

While the author has made every effort to provide accurate telephone numbers and Internet addresses and prices at the time of first printing, neither the publisher, The Stonesong Press, LLC, or the author, assumes any responsibility for errors or for changes that occur after publication.

The author, The Stonesong Press, LLC, and the publisher specifically disclaim any liability, loss, or risk, incurred as a consequence, directly or indirectly of the use and application of any of the contents of this book.

ATRIA BOOKS

A Division of Simon & Schuster, Inc.
1230 Avenue of the Americas
New York, NY 10020

Copyright © 2011 by Little Professor Productions, LLC, and
The Stonesong Press, LLC

First Atria Books edition February 2011
A Stonesong Press Book

ATRIA BOOKS and colophon are trademarks of Simon & Schuster, Inc.

Photography by Stephen Sullivan
CHANEL product photos courtesy of CHANEL
Other photo credits are on page 198.
Spanx Swimsuit sizing chart courtesy of Spanx

For information about special discounts for bulk purchases, please contact Simon & Schuster Special Sales at 1-866-506-1949 or business@simonandschuster.com.

The Simon & Schuster Speakers Bureau can bring authors to your live event. For more information or to book an event, contact Simon & Schuster Speakers Bureau at 1-866-218-3049 or vist our website at www.simonspeakers.com.

Designed by Vertigo Design NYC and produced by The Stonesong Press

Manufactured in the United States of America

10 9 8 7 6 5 4 3 2 1

Library of Congress Cataloging-in-Publication Data

Goodman, Amy E.
  WEAR THIS, TOSS THAT : Hundreds of Fashion and Beauty Swaps That Save Your Looks, Save Your Budget, and Save You Time / Amy E. Goodman.
      pages cm
  1. Clothing and dress. 2. Women's clothing. 3. Fashion. 4. Beauty, Personal. I. Title.
  TT507.G588 2011
  646.4'04--dc22
                                                                          2010047584

ISBN 978-1-4391-8441-7
ISBN 978-1-4391-8443-1 (ebook)

For my darling Fiona and Rowan—
and the privilege of being your mom—
my family, who holds me up to touch my
dreams, and Michael, my love

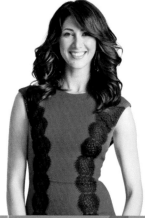

contents

PART ONE
fashion

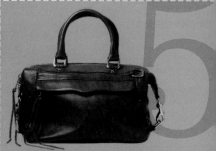

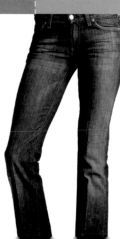

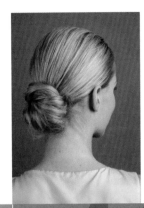

PART
TWO
beauty

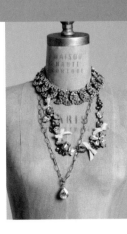

introduction

It *costs* us not to look our best. There, I said it. That's the premise of my fashion philosophy. Every day—believe it or not—clothes can be a saving grace. Here's a case in point: Four months after giving birth to my first child, I had a job interview with a major women's magazine. The night before, I stood in front of the mirror. My tummy still popped, my breasts swelled full, and my softened body felt suspended between my full-term pregnancy clothes on one side of my closet and the now seemingly "miniature" pre-baby clothes on the other. (I mean, *how* did I *zip up* pants that currently stopped at my thighs? Weep.)

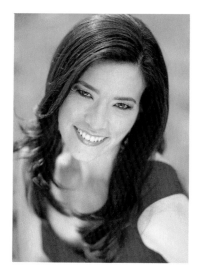

I needed clothes to deliver on so many levels: accommodate my new chest, rein in my new curves…and overcome my lack of confidence. My immediate need was professional, but I still wanted an outfit that could multi-task—one that I could wear from the boardroom to lunch with the girls (and preferably breastfeed in later!).

My final selection was a V-neck wrap dress, which highlighted my waist, gave me a lovely hourglass figure, and kept the chest in check. The deep blue hue slimmed and a diamond pattern detracted from my tummy and made me less self-conscious instantly. Though I felt unsettled and uncharacteristically nervous as I walked into the interview thinking about my newborn, one of three interviewers said, "She just had a baby! Doesn't she look fabulous?"

I got an offer. This wasn't the first time fashion had saved me.

The bottom line is that we *all* need to look good. *All* the time.

WHEN WE **DON'T** DRESS, IT **COSTS** US

- job opportunities
- positive first impressions
- respect
- confidence and self-worth
- dates
- dollars…lots of dollars

We work hard for our money and then toss it away when we fail to wear what we have or buy things we really shouldn't. A rock-bottom price doesn't make a pukey color prettier, a tight-fitting gown looser, or a neon shade less bright.

Packing your closet with clothes you don't wear is equivalent to stocking your refrigerator with foods you don't eat. Sounds absurd, doesn't it?

Thinking of fashion and beauty in terms of value (aside from the price tag) can be complex: easy enough to digest *in theory,* though a little tough to get kicking in reality.

Why is this? Because closets, clothes, fashion…for most people they're something to tackle another day. Until several days later (and several years later) you realize there's a lot you don't like about what you're wearing and you wonder how that happened.

Regardless of what life stage you find yourself in while reading this book (job seeker, newlywed, new mother, divorced, or retired), you need to get dressed—and you need to look phenomenal.

You need fashion answers faster than pronto.

My mission is to help you regain control of your closet by simplifying the choices. I do this rack by rack, piece by piece. Almost instantly, you'll learn what works, what doesn't, and why. Being able to reach into your closet every morning and emerge with options you love is liberating. It means that you have conquered this corner of your world, saving you time and money and affording you opportunities. When so often we don't have power over other areas of our lives—work, relationships, obligations, expectations—reclaiming your wardrobe is a gift you give back to yourself.

up-styling vs. downsizing

When I was younger, I was the kind of girl who enjoyed dressing up. I've always appreciated what fashion has to offer. I was then and am now the one who overdresses for an occasion. As a regular contributor for shows like *Today* and *The View*, and with an editorial career in women's magazines, I'm encouraged to be creative with my personal style and it's acceptable for me to show up with a jeweled Indian *bindi* in the middle of my forehead simply because I think it rocks. Naturally, my friends write me off as the one who always looks put together because of my line of work. But—dare I say—not all magazine editors have style in the same way that not all bank executives dress conservatively.

It's precisely because I like to experiment and switch up what I wear that I have a problem with how we Americans dress. We seem to be obsessed with "comfort clothes." We've adopted the jeans-T-shirt-sneakers look as if it were a national uniform. While dressing down can be entirely stylish, sadly, we define "comfort clothes" as ill-fitting pants, shapeless shirts, and please—don't even get me started on the sweats.

Generally, we turn to clothes as things to throw on and just get us through another day.

What happens then? We glare in the mirror (or avoid it altogether) and take issue with the reflection. Our clothes don't fit. The two pairs of shoes we alternate every other day because they don't hurt are worn out. We look at our closets and wish for a surprise visit from a celebrity stylist. Our hair has been cut and colored the same way for the past five years and we look tired, oh so tired. Some caked eye shadow palettes have followed us from college. The last updo? A ponytail.

As a Japanese-American, I often travel to Tokyo where, if you hop on the subway, you find men in crisp, tailored suits, women with the latest layered tresses, grandmothers dressed to the nines, and students sporting quirky interpretations of the hottest looks. New Yorkers have the same vibe: people dressing to celebrate clothes and showcasing their personal taste. It's energizing. It's exciting. Confidence abounds.

Being surrounded by fashion in motion makes you want to downright… dress up.

So how come so many American women go on fashion furloughs?

1. **I hate my body right now. Why bother?** For the very reason that you deserve to look fantastic no matter your shape or age—20s, 30s, 40s, 50s, 60s, and beyond. As we mature, our bodies play tricks on us. We expand and con-

tract. We flatten and thin. We have a baby or two or three (the belly button is never quite the same, is it?). Even when we do manage to hit the gym, our muscles may firm but our post-childbirth or 40-something skin may still sag. Finally, we've got wrinkles to remind us of the sun-scorching years of our youth.

This book can trump your body's tricks. I acknowledge women's changing appearance and strip down dressing essentials so that you no longer need to hide behind your clothes. I offer **save-me** styling tips that accentuate your body's strengths and the current life stage of your skin. It's the instant boost you need to reclaim your looks.

2. **I don't have the time.** Sure you do. The issue may be putting in the initial hours to get the clothes you really want. With that in mind, I spell out how to sort through the clothes you have, take inventory of what you need, and build upon what you've got to create a winning wardrobe. Before you know it, you'll be throwing an ensemble together in a flash and looking fresh and fabulous every day. Think of this as an investment that will save time in the long run.

3. **Clothes are complicated.** That's right, sister. Trying to figure out what fits and what doesn't is a long labor of love that can last a lifetime as our bodies morph over the years. My goal is to show you easy fashion swaps, hanger by hanger, one piece at a time.

Once you get the basics down, I'll show you how to take it to the next level with fun details that speak to your personal style.

I've done the homework, so you'll be the expert: at the dress department, jeans table, suit section, shoe racks, cosmetics counter, haircare shelves, and more.

4. **Money is tight these days.** I hear you, and so do designers. That's why many of them are developing budget-friendly lines and distributing them through mass merchants for easy access. Clothes are actually more affordable than ever.

I will decode what you really need to construct a fashionable wardrobe and give you a wealth of ideas about where to shop and save money. Did you know there is a web site that will send you an alert when an item you're eyeing—let's say it's a flirty ruffled shirt from J. Crew—goes on sale? Or that you can get cash back at your favorite stores by shopping through a particular source? A recent Consumer Expenditures survey by the U.S. Department of Labor found that a 2.5-person family making $63,000 before taxes spends nearly $2,000 on apparel and nearly $600 on beauty/personal care annually. I think those numbers are a conservative estimate, but regardless, we need to make every one of those dollars count. Whether shopping in the mall or on the Internet, I'll steer you toward the best deals when paying full price is not an option.

5. **I happen to like casual!** Of course you do! Trust me, I do too. I'm not one to go to the gym in dress pants and heels. But there is a snazzy way to wear casual. I'll explain how to find jeans that fit figures of all types (Chapter 2) and show you tops that'll make you sizzle in Chapter 1. (I have more classic options, too.) Before you know it, your "casual safari" will go from bland and drapey to sophisticated and sharp. You'll become queen of your own fashion jungle. My goal is to get you to rethink everyday dressing. I want you to roar, "I never knew casual could look so chic! I never knew this could be so easy!"

who is this book for?

I'm here to share all I know with fellow busy women, regardless of age, lifestyle, location, or fashion IQ. This book is for those who want to wake up their look and shake off under-dressing *without* having to categorize their body as a fruit, vegetable, or geometric form. (Am I shaped like a pear? An eggplant? An inverse triangle?) Yes, good fit is essential, and we'll talk about it plenty, but I've never understood the value of buying a book that defines every body type or identifies every body problem, thus leaving you with only one chapter—or worse, a few pages—that are relevant to you.

Perhaps your body is and has been the same size since you were 18. For the rest of us (raise your hands, majority!), our shapes have changed over the years, whether or not our clothes have kept up with us.

Perhaps you're still trying to squeeze into your old "skinny" jeans, hiding a bit of belly after having a baby or hitting a certain age, or redefining your style as you re-enter the workforce. The key is to no longer hide our figures based on where we've been or where we *think* we're headed. We need clothes for *now* and we need to switch things up because, like any good stock, investing in ourselves pays off.

why me? because i get it

I'm not a fashionista. I grew up in a rural part of northern California, where my earliest fashion memories include my mother's handmade and matching mother-daughter dresses (she was Kanga, I was Roo) and my multi-pocketed cargos for scaling trees in my backyard. As a preteen, I navigated the fashion-forward 1980s with my nine-year-old mentality: jelly bracelets, jelly shoes, a can of AquaNet (for teased bangs, of course), and glow-in-the-dark neon. I watched with my good-girl mouth agape as Madonna single-handedly made lingerie a daytime staple.

Although I attended college on both coasts—Los Angeles and New York City—and my work is in big cities, I currently reside in a suburb of Washington, D.C., and juggle (don't we all?) my roles as wife, mother, daughter, friend, and worker bee. I type these pages pregnant with my second child, on my bed between 9 p.m. and 2 a.m.—my quietest and most productive hours. I call sources on Bluetooth in my car, where my toddler daughter unfailingly chimes in at full volume. As a journalist I cover fashion, beauty, and lifestyle, while shopping the latest sales at CVS, Target, and Loehmann's—and I clip coupons from Saturday circulars to save on sandwich bags.

It is an abundant and multitasking life. Recently, I hosted a forty-person mother-child brunch where assorted muffins, waffles, and coffee cake were served. A friend took one look at my crumb-covered floor and exclaimed, "Better call your house-keeper!" (Save the phone call: You're looking at her.) People also assume I have a nanny. Nannies must be godsends, but we don't have one…at least not yet.

This was written with my friends' everyday questions in mind: Do these shoes go with these capris? Is this skirt length appropriate for my age? How can I make my shrinking boobs look bigger? (Okay…the last question was mine!) What do I wear to a conference in Las Vegas? How do I make sense of organic makeup lines? Where should I shop? We're a single-income household and the kids come first, so how can I look good without spending the milk money?

So no, I'm not a fashion stylist, but I know about fashion. I'm not a makeup artist, but I love dipping my hands in everything beauty. I leave hairstyling to the pros, but I always take note of what they're using. And I've compiled years of curiosity, questioning, and research into this book.

good looks bring big returns in bad times

There isn't a woman alive who hasn't experienced one of those horrific days that drains her emotionally, professionally, or financially. Think about it: The days you can't get out of bed. The job search that makes you feel unskilled. The horrific, unsettling date that left you questioning your character. The news that a loved one is hospitalized, that your teenager is suspended from school, or that your paycheck falls short of this month's bills.

At these crucial moments, dressing down is oh-so-tempting. But it costs us even more. It makes us fall into habits that are counterproductive. When did wearing pajamas all day help you get out of bed? When did not brushing your hair better prepare you to face the outside world?

Looking good can jolt you with self-generated power. It can shift your paradigm when things aren't looking up, so you feel stronger.

This is supported in findings by the 2010 Gamma Beauty Study (conducted by Research Solutions), in which nine out of ten women ages 18 to 64 said makeup can make you feel more confident and that this confidence extends to a positive self-image.

In fairness, I've put this philosophy to the test. Late one night I got a call that I had been let go from a job. The news hit me when I least expected it, without warning and with dirty dinner dishes getting crusty in the sink. Though I was told it wasn't about me, it certainly didn't feel that way. I was thoroughly and utterly shell-shocked.

In the days that followed and, because I'm a creature of habit, I continued to dress as if I was prepping for work, applying my makeup as if I had someplace to go, even though I would have a meltdown and cry thirty minutes later. Sitting in bedclothes would've made me ambivalent. I gave myself some time to "mourn," as I called it (I did mention the bawling, right?), but then I dusted off the résumé and started making calls. Within three months, I'd landed another dream job.

At that time, I could've easily gone down a path of self-loathing (picture *Friends* reruns, unanswered e-mails, and bags of Baked Lay's Potato Crisps), but my physical routine of dressing and maintaining my exterior kept me in check when my interior needed it most.

Armed with clothes and accessories that work and fresh makeup options, anyone can pull off the greatest of deceptions. That's another dividend of fashion and beauty: They are ideal cover-ups for the particularly tough days or nights.

why this journey now?

In the beginning, I talked about what a dressy girl I am. One reason for that—aside from my mother's obsession with dresses for her only daughter—was my early exposure to fashion. My grandmother, a first-generation Japanese-American, was a seamstress (she still sews at 88!) from the moment her ship landed in this country. She subscribed to the best fashion magazines ("This the latest in Paris!" she'd exclaim), which her society clientele flipped through as they streamed in and out of her house for fittings. Luxurious fabrics pouring out of Britex bags from San Francisco, half-cut muslins, fitting forms, straight pins between her lips and precariously littering the floor…these were all a part of visiting Grandma Peggy's house. So I was spoiled. If I bought something at a store, she would tailor fit it to my body, and she custom-made numerous gowns for me. Perched on the arm of her sofa (since the cushions offered no sitting space, being stacked high with sewing supplies and pattern packages scribbled with measurements) is where my fashion education began.

I report deeply and write passionately, knowing that we all bring our unique experiences and bodies to the table. While I personally abhor harem pants, some of you out there swear by them (along with the one runway model from Russia who wears them perfectly). For that matter, fashion wouldn't be fashionable without change and evolution and opinion. Though I've tried to make the WEAR and TOSS fashion choices crystal clear regardless of trends, nothing I've written is an absolute: A TOSS is not a TOSS if it truly works for you. (Make sure a discerning friend heartily agrees and that it's not your stubbornness holding out.) What I do hope to offer are general guidelines, formulated with the best possible intent, as to what works and what doesn't *for most of us*.

People always ask me who the "us" is in this book. Unflinchingly, I say "real women." So let's keep it real. Let's not waste another minute, and let's do this stylishly. Together.

All my love,

[signature]

2:45 a.m.

welcome to your closet

how to use this book

Let's face it, gals: Your closet may be the last thing you think about when you are time-starved, budget-starved, have starving children (*Mom, when's dinner?*), and are overworked and underpaid. But since this is where we keep our clothes, what better place to begin?

In Part One, I have organized the chapters like sections of your closet: from top rack (shirts and sweaters) to bottom rack (pants and skirts), including hanging racks (dresses, suits, and coats), shoe racks, and shelves, drawers, and boxes for accessories (handbags, belts, and jewelry). Then, in Part Two, we bop over to the bathroom to review skincare, makeup, and hair, because a cleaned-up beauty routine is the essential finishing touch to your total look.

The phrase **save-me** is one you've already read and one I'll use throughout the book. A **save-me** functions like a life preserver in either keeping you buoyant as a basic staple, or rescuing you in the case of a fashion emergency. Either way, you'll want a lot of **save-me's** in your life! (I'm afloat because of them.)

WEAR THIS, TOSS THAT! is designed as a reference book to *use*, read repeatedly, and store on your closet shelf for quick consultation. To make the info digestible, I approach fashion choices hanger by hanger, piece by piece. Look for plenty of fun facts sprinkled throughout (**Body Shop, Break This Rule!, Style to Go, Ever Wonder…**) and these recurring **FASHION SIDEBARS**, jam-packed with insider secrets.

AGE ALERT: age-appropriate pointers—the good, the bad, and the downright wrong

BEST BETS: regardless of price, the absolute go-to resource that delivers

DITCH IT: additional items to toss and why, and what to avoid because of body type (thick arms, muffin-top waist, etc.)

IT'S A STEAL: great deals, good prices, best in show for every rack, shelf, and drawer in your closet

MATCH POINT: the dos and don'ts of pairing up ensembles to create a winning or losing look. Here, too, you'll find **SHINING MOMENT:** advice on pairing jewelry with a given look or clothing item

OUTSOURCING/INSOURCING: tailoring tips and other unexpected ways to save big bucks on what's already hanging in your closet

RAISING THE BAR: styling secrets that take an ordinary item to extraordinary

BEHIND THE SEAMS: insider information about fashion

SALE SUCKERS: what not to buy and common mistakes made in purchasing items you don't need

SHAPE SAVER: A-list lingerie, shapewear, and styling suggestions (for lifting and smoothing) for different items of clothing

SOLE MATES: great shoes to pair with various styles of pants, skirts, and dresses

TEMPERATURE FALLING/TEMPERATURE RISING: advice on what to wear for different weather/climates

And for your beauty shelves and drawers, there are tailored **BEAUTY SIDEBARS**.

APPLY THIS: application techniques

THE SCOOP: invaluable beauty factoids about makeup that you should know

BEST BETS: the best in show for beauty items and hair techniques, regardless of price

DITCH IT: additional items to toss and why

IT'S A STEAL: great deals and good prices on quality must-haves

SPOTLIGHT ON HUE: color notes

TRICKS OF THE TRADE: insights from makeup and hair mavens who know

the essential go-to fashion & beauty wardrobe

Admit it: At one point or another, we have what I call "closet case syndrome," where we can't stand to look at our clothes, let alone wear them. It might be a few dated or well-worn pieces that make us wince, or an entire wardrobe we want to swap. It's that moment when we walk away, shake our head, and wonder: Can I rescue what I wore yesterday from the hamper?

Take a step back from the laundry basket.

I trust your intelligence, and you should too. We simply need to organize our fashion thoughts.

In this section, I outline The Fashion Essentials—an extremely selective thirty-piece clothing and thirty-piece accessory wardrobe, followed by The Beauty Essentials that will keep you looking fabulous from head to toe. These are the basics across every clothing and accessory category that can be mixed and matched repeatedly. (This is important: When the dry cleaning is out, you'll still have these staples to turn to in a pinch.) Yes, The Essentials are the bare bones—nothing less and nothing more.

Next to each Essential, such as **4 Shirts**, you'll see a page number that sends you to the precise chapter to see several examples in action. Essentially, you need at least two button-down shirts and two blouses. But of those two blouses, it's entirely up to you whether you choose a ruffled number or a sleeveless cut or a printed blouse. This is where you get to exercise your fashion freedom to select a choice that suits your personality, your body, and your specific needs.

Since I want to maximize your options, within each chapter, under OTHER MUST HAVES, you'll find tips for the trickier aspects of what to buy beyond the basics. This is where you can really be creative, adding to The Essentials to give your fashion and beauty wardrobe true character that, at its core, represents who you are.

But let's not get ahead of ourselves. Without a thread of excess, **THE ESSENTIAL FASHION AND BEAUTY WARDROBE** should look like this:

fashion essentials

the 30 clothes you can't live without

4 shirts *(top rack, page 2)*
+ 2 button-down shirts (make one neutral—black or gray, white or cream, brown or tan)
+ 2 blouses

2 stylish Ts *(top rack, page 2)*
+ 1 short or long sleeve
+ 1 tank

5 sweaters *(top rack, page 2)*
+ 3 neutral sweaters
+ 2 colorful sweaters

6 pants *(bottom rack, page 26)*
+ 3 trousers
+ 3 jeans (one of each for play, date night, work)

3 skirts *(bottom rack, page 26)*
+ 2 pencil or A-line skirts
+ 1 full/long skirt or short skirt

4 dresses *(hanging rack, page 54)*
+ 2 work/day dresses
+ 1 little black dress
+ 1 colorful cocktail dress

3 suits *(with pants or skirt; hanging rack, page 54)*
+ 1 black
+ 1 other neutral tone
+ 1 color

3 coats *(hanging rack, page 54)*
+ 1 trench
+ 1 fitted blazer
+ 1 three-quarter-length

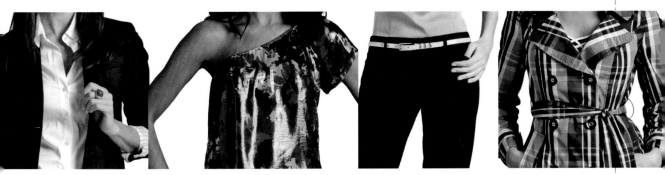

the 30 instant-update accessories

9 shoes *(shoe rack, page 84)*

+ 3 heels
+ 3 flats
+ 2 boots (one heeled, one flat)
+ 1 stylish sneaker

5 bags *(top shelf, page 100)*

+ 2 neutrals (make one of them black or brown)
+ 1 color
+ 1 tote
+ 1 evening bag

2 belts *(make one of them neutral; accessory drawer, page 110)*

+ 1 medium-width belt
+ 1 narrow belt

jewelry *(accessory box, page 120)*

+ 2 pairs chandelier earrings
+ 3 pairs stud earrings
+ 2 short necklaces
+ 2 long necklaces
+ 2 bangles and/or cuffs
+ 2 watches (one leather band, one link)
+ 1 cocktail ring

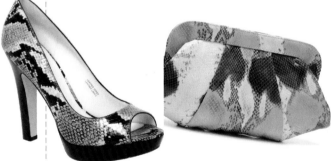
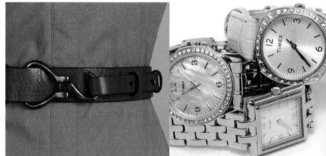

beauty essentials

basic skincare
(skincare shelf, page 132)

+ cleanser
+ mist
+ facial exfoliator
+ lip balm and lip exfoliator
+ 2 moisturizers (day and night)
+ eye cream
+ sunscreen
+ anti-aging masques and/or treatments, as age-appropriate

must-have makeup
(cosmetics drawer, page 146)

+ makeup primer
+ concealer
+ 2 foundations (one for winter, one for summer)
+ facial powder
+ 2 blushes (one for winter, one for summer)
+ bronzer

+ brow liner or powder
+ eyeliner
+ eye shadow color palette with light and dark shades and highlighter
+ mascara
+ 4 lipsticks (two for winter, two for summer)
+ lip gloss
+ eyelash curler
+ tweezers
+ set of makeup brushes
+ matte oil blotting papers

cure-all hair solutions
(haircare shelf, page 170)

+ shampoo
+ conditioner
+ deep conditioning treatment
+ styling products for hair type
+ hair dryer
+ curling iron
+ flat iron

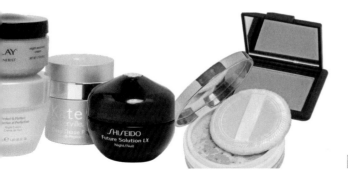
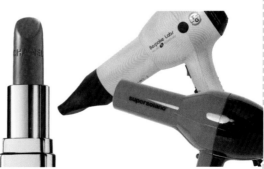

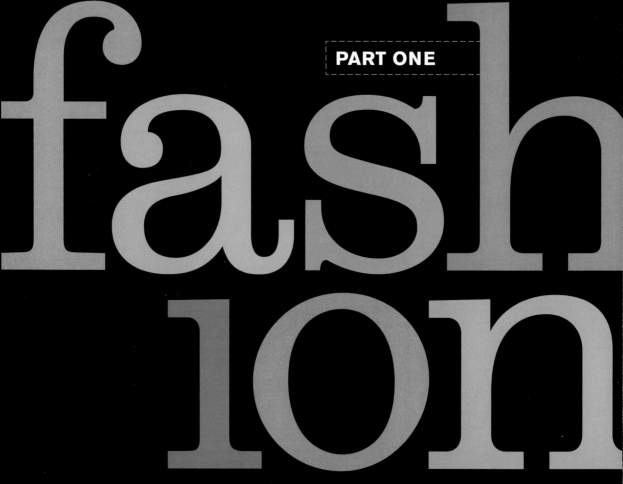

PART ONE

fash
ion

Stand in front of your closet and take stock. Chances are you have a lot of clothes…more clothes than you ever wear, more clothes than you feel good about, more clothes than you realize you own. Whether you live to shop or shy away from it, we all have clothes that never see the light of day because they…

1. don't fit

2. aren't stylish

3. need tailoring

4. are long forgotten under an avalanche of seriously so-so options

Like anything else that involves storage, closets seem to accumulate items all on their own. Our need to organize them only arises when we have extra time on our hands (anybody got some… anybody?) or when we move and we're forced to take inventory, which is what we're going to do right now. Take out the clothes you haven't worn in two to three years and sort them into four piles.

wear clothes in pristine condition that you still love and plan to wear

maybe clothes you feel ambivalent about keeping

toss clothes that are in bad condition or hopelessly outdated and headed for the garbage

charity clothes in good condition that can be donated

Next, pull out clothes that have stains or need repair and place that pile in a bag to take to the tailors or cleaners the next chance you get.

Listen ladies, we all know parting with clothes is *painful*. We're attached to what we wear. But if you aren't using something, why keep someone else (in the case of the charity pile) from wearing it now?

If you are still on the fashion fence about your "maybes" or cannot even commit an item to a pile, don't throw in the hanger! Read on, and I'll show you what to WEAR and what to TOSS.

top rack :

shirts & sweaters

wear

basic shirt

The quintessential shirt: tailored, feminine, and fitted, made with stretch fabric for easy movement. The workmanship presents an overall crisp feeling.

+ Fabric that smoothly contours to your body
+ Seams that lie flat
+ A shirt with darts that tailor the bust and torso
+ A collar that doesn't under- or overwhelm the shape of your face
+ Buttons that don't pull—no peep shows here!
+ A length that proportionally flatters, hitting between the waist and hips for most torsos and below the hip line for those with wide hips
+ Catchy details…a neck tie or waist tie
+ Interesting patterns such as lines, dots, lace

IT'S A STEAL

A fresh and rockin' U.K. import, Topshop (www.us.topshop .com) wows crowds with its darling shirts and tops while offering a welcome respite from jaw-dropping prices.

RAISING THE BAR

Hey non-shirt-tuckers…sensitive about your tummy? Listen up. If your shirt hits the top of your pants or hangs one or two inches longer, leave it untucked. If it's longer, falling beyond your hipbone, suck it up and tuck. Add a belt for definition. (See Chapter 6 for more on belts.)

SHAPE SAVER

Until the ultimate back-flab-eliminating exercise comes along, there's Shapeez The Shortee Unbelievabra ($75; www.unbelievabra.com) a bra with a built-in rear shapewear tank to hold the twins in and keep your back from having boobs too.

AGE ALERT

Button up all the way up if you're going geek or recreating the Victorian Era. Otherwise, leave the top buttons undone and create a youthful look by topping with a vest

or a cropped jacket…additions that still offer a "buttoned up" feeling of containment.

6

The number of months after which you need new bras—or sooner if your weight fluctuates

- A shirt that's too tight around the bra
- Fabric that clings to your back fat, love handles, breasts
- Seams that pop up or snake unevenly down your shoulders or sides
- Arm holes that are too small
- A shirt that is so worn it's sheer
- Uncuttable loose threads (they unravel into holes when snipped)
- A length that has shrunken to reveal belly or, conversely, is stretched long and shapeless
- Colors faded from washing
- Cheesy souvenir T-shirts or ones with offensive phrases

basic shirt

A poorly fitting top with buttons that pull on the torso, causing wrinkles.

BASIC SHIRT

top rack : shirts

age alert

Fretting about flabby arms? Avoid sleeves that are short on coverage. This means sleeve-less styles and cap sleeves that cut off your biceps at their widest point, turning arms into little sausages (take it from me, I've made the mistake on national TV!). Half, three-quarter, and long sleeves that flutter are your best bet.

sale suckers

If you constantly pull your shirt in any direction, it doesn't fit. Consider buttons that are closer together (fewer gaps).

Opt for combination fabrics with stretch to give you room to groove. Don't load up on skin-tight, stretch-only fabrics (Lycra, spandex, jersey)—not even if you are a rock-hard sensation.

ditch it

A bad shirt that makes you look bigger? No thanks. Avoid shimmering fabrics (they shine like high beams, dispersing light in all directions), hori-zontal stripes (they widen by drawing eyes east and west), and shirts with too much detailing (they add bulk).

insourcing

Hate to iron but detest looking disheveled? Brooks Brothers Non-Iron Shirts with a touch of stretch come to the rescue. They're available in three cuts: tailored, fitted, and classic. At nearly $90 each they are pricey, but being able to put on a shirt that looks freshly pressed, com-plete with darts, straight out of the *dryer*? Priceless (www.brooksbrothers.com, 800-274-1815).

wear

A V-neck wrap shirt with a tailored hem, a belted waist, and a neck-line that shows some skin.

other must HAVES

+ **Sewn wrap shirts with side zipper**, that allows for ease of entry, exit, and wear
+ **Short sleeve wrap shirts**
+ Standard **V-neck shirts**, tailored to the body for a more casual option

RAISING THE BAR

Universally flattering, **save-me** wrap shirts let you custom-fit the shirt to your body, high-lighting your chest, showing a little skin, and accentuat-ing your waist. Look for chic side ties that lie flat and don't bulk the waist. (Back ties are okay, but get ready for some discomfort if you lean back.)

SHINING MOMENT

This is the quintessential V-neck shirt, and it deserves a splashy statement necklace to showcase its incredible neckline. For gorgeous, intri-cate South American–inspired pieces that shine in either gold or silver, try an Eva Longoria favorite, Claudia Lobao jewelry (www.claudialobao.com).

SHAPE SAVER

If your neckline is still too re-vealing, try the Boob Tube by Miss Oops, a lace bandeau that offers perfect coverage beneath any over-revealing V-neck without added bulk. This **save-me** helped conceal my ever-expanding chest during my latest pregnancy. Avail-able in beige, white, or black, $25; www.missoops.com.

BEHIND THE SEAMS

Flowy fabrics such as silk, rayon, and cotton blends fabulously hug the body for a polished fit. Stiffer fabrics work better for a larger frame: They smooth over curves for a streamlined silhou-ette. I prefer a length that goes just beyond my hips. Never tuck the wrap shirt.

An un-adjustable, sewn-in "wrap" shirt that is made of stiff, unyielding fabric in a blah color with knotting that adds bulk to your bust.

other must LOSE

- **Overly ruffled wrap shirts** that lose the clean lines this look provides

- **Kimono-style wrap shirts** that cause the neck to disappear

- **Shirts with wrap ties** that go around the stomach several times before knotting in a bow

ditch it

While a wrap shirt usually fits all, some details don't: Extra-wide collars detract from the stunning décolletage of this style and make your shoulders look unending; ties that are extra long bulk up your waist when they are bowed or knotted.

sale suckers

A poorly fitting sewn wrap shirt is nearly impossible to get into because your head must pass through the narrowly sewn waist. Once on, cleavage may spill out or underwhelm the preconstructed neckline of the top. If you pull at the neck or feel that the gathered portion in the middle adds thickness, try a tie-on wrap shirt and note the difference.

insourcing

Don't wear a wrap shirt by itself if too much skin is exposed. Layer a decorative camisole or vintage tank underneath so that it extends just beyond the shirt's hem, and tie the top less tightly if you feel squeezed. Avoid bulky blouses and medium-weight sweaters under wraps.

wear

A sophisticated tank in a vibrant color with ruffles that sweetly frame the neckline.

other must HAVES

+ **Long sleeve pintucked blouses** for crisp fall nights

+ **Ruffled halters** that are ultra-feminine and flirty, showing off your shoulders

+ **Ruffled tunics** with a body-slimming cut

RAISING THE BAR

Ruffles come in all shapes and sizes: as darts up and down a shirt and around the scoop of a neck, as sleeves, or as frilly details. In general, clustered ruffles *add* shape—the impression of a chest if you don't have one or feminine curves to boyish hips. Too girlie? Choose a top with ruffled sleeves to capture the look without going overly frou-frou.

BEST BETS

Romeo & Juliet Couture is my go-to brand for casual clothes in girlie cuts. They put ruffles on tiered racer-back tanks, basic blouses, keyhole-banded tunics, dresses, and skirts. Check out www.romeoandjulietcouture. com for styles, also available discounted at www.bluefly.com.

MATCH POINT

A gossamer ruffle shirt is certainly sexy, but it's also see-through. It's best paired with a solid-color jacket or a boyfriend blazer to give it some balance. Always wear a bra and undergarments in the same color as the shirt.

SHAPE SAVER

Emporio Armani's Seriously Sexy Underwear Collection makes a stunning black slip camisole with a built-in demi-cup bra, perfect for wearing under a see-through blouse, for about $100; www.emporioarmani.com.

High-density ruffles that jam together like bumper-to-bumper traffic, an additional tie that chokes the neck, and thick cuffs that add to a heavy, busy look.

other must LOSE

- **Baby-doll ruffled shirts** with an A-line cut that make you look pregnant

- **Prints + ruffles** rarely jive as a digestible match, particularly against bold plaids

- **Diagonal ruffles** that run across the tummy, adding unwanted girth

ditch it

Too many ruffles running up and down your shirt is not a look for the well endowed… it overly showcases the chest, where you and your girls alone make enough of a statement.

age alert

Ruffles are classic and add elegance to any given look. That said, the best option as we age is to keep our silhouette simple. Where tiered ruffles only look good on the select few (perhaps the squeakingly young), a single ruffle plait down the front of a blouse flatters nearly everyone by creating length.

sale suckers

If a shirt sports ruffles on only one lapel, take a close look at yourself in the dressing room mirror. Chances are you'll look off balance and ready to fall over!

wear

A top with billowing sleeves—known as blouson—this blouse is comfortable yet defined and has details like metallic buttons and slight gathers around the neckline.

other must HAVES

+ Cotton **peasant tops**
+ **Sleeveless versions** with drawstrings at or below your natural waist
+ **Ethnic blouses** with hand-sewn embroidery
+ **Fluttery lace woven tops** that give a breezy feel

IT'S A STEAL

When Jovovich-Hawk designed for Target, I was among the first to snatch up a versatile, cream-colored blouson-sleeve top for $24.99. For affordable designers with an ethereal and romantic approach to blouses, take a look at www.jovovich-hawk.com, www.joie.com, and www.ellamoss.com. A new offshoot of Forever21 called Love21offers blouson-sleeve tops with sweet detailing at around $30; www.forever21.com.

AGE ALERT

The blouson-sleeve top hides unflattering arms by camoflauging them with a touch of poof.

MATCH POINT

In keeping with its free-spirited shape, the blouson-sleeve blouse should almost always be untucked. Your bottom half, therefore, *must* be fitted. Straight-leg jeans, tailored trousers, or a skinny skirt fit the bill. Avoid a full skirt that will make you one big mushroom on top and bottom.

RAISING THE BAR

We automatically think of peasant-inspired shirts as white, but try a blouson-sleeve blouse in an unexpected color like yellow, red, purple, or navy with feminine details (like black lace on white or embroidery), or a more modern, abstract print.

other must LOSE

- **Oversized flannels**
- **Super crinkled cottons**
  for a sloppy, disheveled look
- **Drapey knit pullovers**

Bat wings (or attached sleeves) are best suited for those who want to disguise heavy arms and a thick waist, but this pirate-style top offers little justice to any maiden.

BODY SHOP

if your shoulders are:

WIDE

wear tailored sweetheart neckline or U-neck to draw attention to décolletage

toss boat neck, scoop neck, thick straps, and wide lapels

NARROW

wear sleeveless, puffy sleeves, wide collars, and wide scoop necks

toss raglan sweaters, crew necks, dropped sleeves, spaghetti straps, and halters

ditch it

Anyone who loves *Pirates of the Caribbean* has a distant fantasy of donning a billowy white blouse. Well, resist. A bit of extra fabric is allowed, but get too unstructured and I fear you'll blow away with the next storm.

it's a steal

Newport News offers some unexpected ruffled and flounce-sleeved options that steady and steer the finer points of this pirate look for women (www.newport-news.com). Their front-tie silk blouses offer the freedom of this style while remaining presentable options for work.

temperature falling

Don't bunch this flowy top under a structured coat or blazer—they're both way too formal. Instead, go with a more casual leather jacket that will allow the blouse to peep out a few inches beneath it.

wear

A tastefully revealing one-shoulder top with a streamlined neck that lies flat—in a metallic print for fashion fun.

other must HAVES

+ **One-shoulder tops** in solid colors for more flattery

+ **On-the-shoulder scoop necks** for showing just the right amount of skin

RAISING THE BAR

This is the ultimate solution for a broad-shouldered broad who still wants some northern exposure. While an off-the-shoulder scoop neck or strapless style overemphasizes the shoulders, an asymmetrical line divides and conquers the space between them.

SHAPE SAVER

Don't even try to wear a strap bra with this number: You'll never be able to hide it. A great strapless bra for the occasion: Maidenform's One Fabulous Fit Strapless Bra with Stay There Power Band and comfy micro-fiber fabric, $31; www.maidenform.com.

MATCH POINT

Balance the flowy nature of this top by pairing it with slim-fit or straight-leg jeans for a tailored lower half. Everything from a stiletto heel to a platform sandal is an ideal choice for your feet, and you can't go wrong with dangling earrings or a draping necklace and/or a stack of thin bracelets.

An off-the-shoulder blouse with a neckline that makes you look too wide on top and too narrow on bottom.

other must LOSE

- **Scoop necks with cap sleeves**, which broaden shoulders *and* create sausage arms

- **Off-the-shoulder, black-and-white animal-print blouses**, where you get lost in the jungle

- **Deeply plunging off-the-shoulder tops** where a breast might flash with one wrong move

age alert
This is *not* the look for someone sensitive about her décolletage. The skin exposure of the neck and chest can further age you, especially if you blush at the sight of protruding bones and wrinkling necks.

ditch it
Attention women with wide shoulders: Run away and don't look back. Because some of these tops double as tunics—extending beyond the hip bone for a long, lean look—they might seem appealing, but they're not worth it when you end up looking like a hockey player on top.

sale suckers
You buy this because you think it's sexy and lets you flash some of the softest skin you've got. Other tops (like the one-shoulder) can offer more sex appeal. This square shape makes you look like a capital T…as in top-heavy.

best bets
For scoop necks in a variety of tasteful dips, from at the neck to below the collarbone, turn to Ann Taylor, (www.anntaylor.com) and LC Lauren Conrad and ELLE, exclusively at Kohl's (www.kohls.com).

wear

top rack : shirts

EMBELLISHED TANK

The ultimate day-to-night top: a fitted tank that has necklaces sewn into the garment or around the neckline. Doff a cardigan and you're ready for Happy Hour.

other must HAVES

+ **Silky tanks** with pailettes (large sequins) on necklines for just the right dose of trend

+ **Cotton tanks** with jeans or cords for casual occasions

+ **Blouson tanks** with ribbed waists for holding and hiding a jiggly tummy

MATCH POINT

Another take on this top is one with attached faux gems. But is being bejeweled too glitzy or heavy for your taste? Sequins offer an alternate way to glam with less weight, and are popping up in daytime looks right now.

BEST BETS

Sweetees offers ultra-comfy tanks with choice embellishments such as large-cut gems, multicolored wooden beads and patterned sequins. See the latest looks at www.mellies.com; purchase at www.shopstyle.com.

SHAPE SAVER

Saggy boobs underneath this top would make this a sinking ship, and visible bra straps are a screaming SOS: Save Our Schnoobies! The best racer-back bra for tank tops is the Wacoal Custom Contours T-Back Bra, $50; www.wacoal-america.com.

AGE ALERT

Who said tanks are only for teens? Sophisticated styles, like those by Simply Vera Vera Wang, can be layered under blazers and add pizzazz at any age…particularly if you have arms to flaunt.

IT'S A STEAL

To keep slipping bra straps in place, try Strap Doctor. Apply this washable, reusable strip of material with its hundreds of microscopic hooks to the underside of your bra strap, with the smooth silicone side facing your skin. It keeps your straps invisible and out of sight ($9.95; www.strapdoctor.com).

BEHIND THE SEAMS

Tank tops evolved from the top of the early bathing suit called the "tank suit," which originated in the 1920s.

14

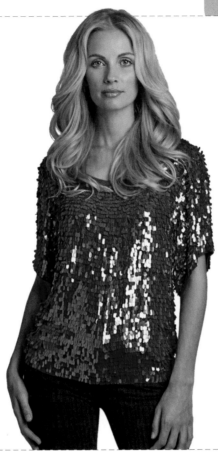

A densely sequined top that refracts light like a disco ball and makes people stop in their tracks—because they are blinded by the bright color.

other must LOSE

- Tops with **poorly sewn sequins** that appear to be scaling off
- **Wide horizontally striped sequined tops** that add visual weight
- **Sequins in overly bold, elaborate patterns** like animal or abstract prints
- **Sequined vests**

shining moment

Pair loads of jewelry with this sparkler and you'll create too many fireworks. Balance is key when working with sequins, so don't go overboard: add some simple earrings, a single splashy cocktail ring, or a bodacious bangle.

sole mates

Bejeweled shoes are too matchy; add a headdress and you're ready for Carnival. Instead, wear neutral-toned shoes that don't scream for attention.

sale suckers

All jewels are *not* the same. Ugly crystals that look pasty will never shine, no matter how you wear them.

best bets

Pick all black or all gray when wearing an all-sequined top. Complementary two-toned styles, like silver and gray or bronze and gold, also work and are truly contemporary, adding depth and dimension. (Look to designers Stella Mc-Cartney and Proenza Schouler for well-executed examples.)

wear

A slimming sweater of medium weight that hits just past the hip, with a V-neck to show some skin, and a mid-length sleeve.

+ A medium-weight fabric that's neither too bulky for a big chest nor too thin for a flat chest

+ A neckline that doesn't crowd your face

+ A belted style if you have a generous bust or hips, to add definition at your waist

+ Unique prints, embroidery, sequins, asymmetrical necklines

+ Details that hide your weaknesses. Flat chested? Look for embellishment around the boobs. Big tummy? Go for a more open neckline to draw attention toward the face

+ Affordable, trendy sweaters from mass retailers to boost your wardrobe for one season

+ A variety of staples: thinner fabrics to layer under a blazer; medium-weight, hand-knitted threads for warmth; standalone twinsets

IT'S A STEAL

My favorite place on earth to load up on sweater basics? UNIQLO. This Japanese import offers seasonal sweaters of every thickness, fabric, and style...including its signature affordable cashmere (www.uniqlo.com).

BEHIND THE SEAMS

The most flattering sweaters show some skin. Think V-necks and scoop necks and go as low as you feel comfortable. (See page 25 "Collars 101" for more on necklines.)

INSOURCING

Pills are a pill—those annoying little fuzz balls collect on a sweater's surface and make it appear old and worn. Invest in a handheld fabric shaver that removes the pills. My favorite is the Surround Air XJ-350 Electric Fabric Shaver, $29.99; www.target.com.

AGE ALERT

When adding a long scarf, drape it around your neck and let it hang freely. A scarf knotted around a high neckline creates a crowded look that instantly ages.

toss

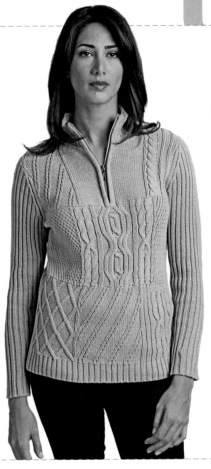

- Heavy appliqués, such as seasonal Christmas trees, pumpkins, autumn leaves, or braided embroidery, that weigh a sweater down

- Any sweater with blinking lights attached to a battery pack

- "Wire hanger" shoulders

- Shapeless sweaters

- Overly fuzzy fabrics like angora that shed

- Thin fabrics that cling to stomach rolls

- Thick fabrics that bunch up under arms or at waist

Overly chunky, overly detailed, heavy knit sweater that makes you look "stuffed" like after Thanksgiving dinner, with an unattractive zip funnel neck.

shape saver
Don't have Madonna's killer biceps? Tres Sleek is an innovative shapewear that compresses sagging arm muscles into place, eliminating the "bingo wing," says creator Lee Ann Stevenson. They're $32 to $51; www.tressleek.com, 800-471-3830.

age alert
A cropped sweater that unveils your tummy is too revealing if you've received your high school diploma. (This can happen with a regular sweater if it's too short and rises high.) Unless you plan on layering underneath *every time*, leave this look to the *Twilight* tweens.

behind the seams
Many women don't realize their sweaters have worn elbows until they are told to look for them and then, wow!, there they are. I had this cashmere purple sweater my grandmother gave me. It had a small moth-eaten hole I thought no one could see. I wore it forever…and honestly, everyone could see it. Don't let this happen to you.

insourcing
Don't dry clean your cashmere, which is a highly delicate, downy wool that comes from the underbelly of a Kashmir goat.

Hand washing is the way to go (and more budget-friendly). Turn the sweater inside out, hand wash in room-temperature water with a wool-cleansing shampoo, then lay flat to dry.

it's a steal
For a green and biodegradable wash that leaves sweaters ultra soft with a fresh cedar scent, try The Laundress, Wool & Cashmere Shampoo, $19; www.thelaundress.com. It's a **save-me** for getting dry-cleaned results at home.

wear

A long cardigan that hits past hips in a deep shade or versatile neutral, with flat pockets, in a medium fabric that hangs gracefully over curves.

other must HAVES

+ **Long, ribbed cardigans** with matching cloth belt ties
+ **Weighty, woven cardigans** of three-quarter length to wear in colder weather
+ **Long pullover sweaters** that hug your silhouette

IT'S A STEAL

For pieces like long, slouchy cardigans, check out Boutique to You (www.boutiquetoyou.com), which celebrates the latest casual fashion of the young celebrity set with direct links for purchasing star-inspired looks. For fun, shop by celeb. With seasonal "blowout" sales, amazing deals abound.

RAISING THE BAR

Long cardigans are super slimming. Typically ending at mid-thigh with a long, uninterrupted vertical line, they hide a wide tush, hips, and generous thighs.

MATCH POINT

For work, button and belt at the waist with a skinny belt. For play, leave unbuttoned with a hipster belt. To reduce bulk, keep your inner layer thin. Do *not* go too wide on the belt: you'll look dowdy.

BODY SHOP

if your neck is:

SHORT

wear V-necks, U-necks, and scoop necks, as low as you feel comfortable

toss crew, cowl, mock, and turtlenecks that shorten a short neck and emphasize a double chin

LONG

wear funnel necks, tie-necks, and turtlenecks

toss long, open shawl collars and deeply plunging V-necks that make your neck look even longer

A super drapey and undefined long-sleeve wrap, in a drab color, that looks more like an airplane blanket than an article of clothing.

other must LOSE

- **Wide-cut, single button knitted cardigans** that add chunk

- **Button-down cardigans** that end with a ruffle right on the hip

- **Cardigans so open** and embellished that they cannot be secured in the front

temperature falling

It's tempting to embrace loads of fabric to avoid freezing, but any sweater that describes itself as a "cocoon" or a "maxi" probably has too much. If a wrap ends at the thickest part of your thigh, the widest part of your buttocks, or—like a short poncho—the bulkiest part of your waist, skip it. These are *not* areas to target, even if you feel toasty warm beneath.

best bets

Have a near-new sweater that you'd like to swap for a different look? A number of sites, like the international www.swapace .com, make even exchanges a snap (a sweater for a sweater without the exchange of cash). Includes simple-to-follow icons and easy posting. And it's all free!

ditch it

People rejoice in wraps because they can effectively hide their tummies without resorting to the suck-it-in method. But the truth is, an oversized wrap makes the attempt too obvious. Look for wraps that offer you shape and are made of thin but warm fabrics like wool, cashmere, or an acrylic blend.

wear

A draped sexy style or a tailored look with flattering ribbing, in a standout fabric with detail such as subtle shine.

other must HAVES

+ **Long, knit sweater coats** cinched with a belt

+ Sweaters with metal clasps or toggle buttons or other **interesting closures** that jazz up a knit

+ **Knitted shrugs** with a slight A-line flair that end at the thinnest part of your waist

BEST BETS

Ever wonder what are the best days to shop online for the *deepest* discounts? In a recent study of 90,000 online purchases by Shop It To Me, Wednesday is the new Friday in terms of best online sale prices for men's clothing, women's accessories, shoes, and intimates. Tuesday is the best day for buying a dress (up to 55 percent off), and Wednesday and Thursday are when retailers put the most new sale items up for grabs.

RAISING THE BAR

A sexy knit is a **save-me** sweater. Wear scoop neck styles to work layered over a thin camisole or tank and cap-sleeve knits with long-sleeve blouses. Then do a Clark Kent quick change and wear it solo as an after-hours staple.

BEST BETS

Go retro with a draped style (in a women's cut, but still made to look like you stole it from your beau's closet), gathered a bit at the hips, with a touch of sparkle in the weave. H&M always updates its oversized knit styles in fall/winter. Use the "create your own style" guide on the store's site to play with sweaters and silhouettes before you buy (www.hm.com/us).

IT'S A STEAL

For the sweetest handmade knitted boleros, wraparound scarves, neck warmers, and shawls, check out New York–based www.deniz03 .etsy.com, where prices range from $22 to $58.

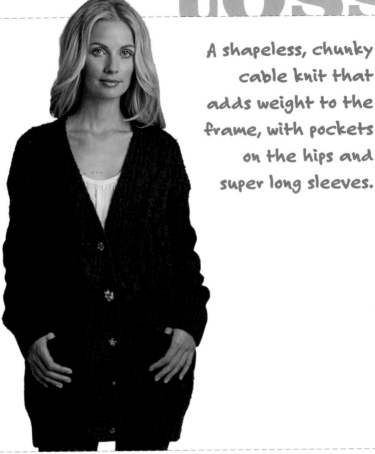

A shapeless, chunky cable knit that adds weight to the frame, with pockets on the hips and super long sleeves.

other must LOSE

- **Knitted turtlenecks** (unless incredibly thin) that overwhelm the face, chest, and chin
- **Chunky sweaters** in an A-line that get wider and thicker toward the hips and tummy
- **Ruffled sweaters** that can add bulk to the chest and upper torso

shape saver

Don't hang a sweater on a hanger until you check out the innovative Precision Hangers ($18.95 to $19.95; www.precisionhangers.com) that stop creases and dimples. Store a chunky knit sweater folded in a drawer or on a shelf.

break this rule!

Thought scarves were only for winter? Wearing cold weather knitted scarves in warm seasons is a growing trend. Another hot move: wearing a lightweight scarf with a coat.

insourcing

A large weave sweater can easily catch and pull—ruined!—by the end of a season. To fix pulled yarn and prolong wear, turn the sweater inside out and use a needle to pull in loose threads.

behind the seams

Chunky sweaters are generally not for those who are well endowed or self-conscious about a thick upper torso or love handles. If you fit one of these descriptions, opt for a more finely milled fabric like merino wool. It has texture and hides imperfections.

72

percentage of people who go out of their way to shop at an outlet mall

wear

An unexpected twinset: pair a contrast trim cardigan with a thin, simple underlying layer that lies flat on the body.

other must HAVES

+ **Twinsets of varying lengths** where the outer cardigan is bolero length and the inner layer is long

+ **Column-shaped, one-button cardigans** that counterbalance hips if you're pear shaped

SHINING MOMENT

Jazz up a twinset with a vintage brooch (placed one or two inches off the neckline to the right or left of center) or a statement necklace atop a boat-neck or a V-neck style. For stunning vintage jewels at super prices, look at www.rustyzipper.com > accessories > jewelry. Or renowned trimming store M&J Trimming has new brooches with old-world glamour, www.mjtrim.com > flower pins & pendants > brooches.

MATCH POINT

Think beyond the perfect pair and separate the twins. The knitted tank or sweater can stand alone in warmer temps and can be paired with long necklaces, while the cardigan can be layered on top of other separates.

RAISING THE BAR

If you cannot find a twinset that appeals, piece together your own version. Colors don't need to match exactly—the top cardigan can be a print while the underneath layer is a solid. The key is to find fabrics that are similar in weight and look.

other must LOSE

— **Twinsets with super high necklines**

— **Twinsets with wavy, striped patterns** that add girth

A twinset in a matchy-matchy print and a cheap synthetic material that both ages and pales your complexion.

BODY SHOP

if your face is:

OVAL OR HEART-SHAPED

wear boat neck—higher neckline brings attention to shoulders and complements the widest variety of long face shapes

toss cowl neck—drapes loosely on the chest, making oval faces look too long and chins on heart-shaped faces too pointy

ROUND

wear scoop neck/shawl collar—open space at chest draws eye up and down to flatter a round face

toss crew neck—round, tight neckline accentuates face's roundness

SQUARE

wear ruffled neck—balances defined bone structure with softness

toss pointed collar—angles overly emphasize square jaw

age alert

Button up. It may feel counterintuitive, but this ensemble works best when you button the outer layer to hide the inner layer. Fastening even the top two buttons makes a chic statement. Leave the bottom two buttons near the waist undone.

sole mates

The worst possible pairing with the traditional twinset would be flat flats (as in boring). Elevate this look with some killer heels in an unexpected color: red, yellow, purple.

ditch it

Because this look is conservative, don't ever pair with a super long skirt. If you are covered up on top, show some skin below. The ultimate match: a pencil skirt.

23

wear

A primo-condition vintage sweater with delicate beading, no stains, a soft, sweet look, and details specific to its time period (this one is from the 1950s).

other must HAVES

+ **Tiny fit vintage cardigans** that you can use as chic cover-ups

+ **Vintage V-neck sweater tops**—same classic shape, why not save money?

+ **Missoni-esque striped '70s sweaters**

IT'S A STEAL

People who know me know I love vintage. It celebrates fashion from another era and brings old-world elegance to modern clothes. Plus, it's green and affordable. What's not to adore? Take the plunge at local vintage shops in your area. True diggers can unearth amazing finds at Salvation Army and Goodwill.

BEST BETS

My favorite contemporary consignment shop, with a ninety-day revolving inventory and twenty-two stores on the East Coast, is Second Time Around (www.secondtime-around.net). For more specific searches (women's vintage clothing > 1960s > cream sweater) use eBay.com for great deals or pricing estimates.

INSOURCING

Do yourself a favor and don't buy subpar vintage—unless you're handy with a needle and thread and are willing to re-stitch fraying embroidery, torn linings, loose buttons, or missing beading. And some issues, like stains and moth holes, will never disappear, even with professional assistance.

ever wonder how consignment shops work?

They typically allow third parties to sell their goods and retain a portion of the profit after sale. They're also an amazing source for all things vintage. Traditionally, items are price-reduced after a certain period of time. For the crème de la crème of online designer consignment, try www.thesnob.net or www.covetshop.com.

other must LOSE

- **College sweatshirts** from your or your *child's* college, worn outside your house
- **Faded sports shirts**—go ahead, get a new jersey in a women's size for game days
- **Oversized rugby shirts**

COLLARS 101

NEHRU Also known as the Chinese collar, the Nehru has a short, standing band that wraps around the neck like a priest's Roman collar. It may have a V or a space in the front.

SHAWL Like a loose shawl wrapped around a neck, this collar has a relaxed, rolled look.

POINTED Crisp pointed ends define this classic collar.

PETER PAN This flat, rounded collar tightly frames the neck and is usually buttoned or closed.

RUFFLED All ruffled up: Ruffled collars are diverse. They can outline a V-neck, fully engulf a blouse from collar to bodice, and/or lie flat to resemble a tuxedo bib.

NOTCHED The notched collar is named for the slitted V on the collar.

PILLOW As it sounds: it is poofy, fluffy, rounded, and often part of down coats.

PORTRAIT A really wide collar, it frames the face like a portrait.

TIE The tie can be high at the neck or loose, like a V-neck, cascading down the front or side of the shirt.

FUNNEL A standing collar around the neck, this collar is not as snug as a turtleneck. It may or may not have overlapping folds. In a coat, it's usually secured with a front zipper.

COWL A super drapey collar that can extend all the way to shoulders, like a collar on Prozac.

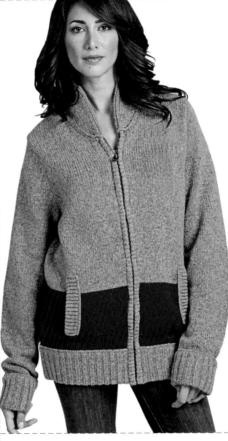

A varsity, sporty, or club cardigan sweater with rugby charm or a thick weave— a remnant from university days that should remain a college memory.

VARSITY

top rack : sweaters

it's a steal

This look was very hot…when you were in school. But if you must wear this style, look for clean lines and a sophisticated color scheme: think nautical. Try Ralph Lauren's reasonably priced Rugby line (www.rugby.com).

ditch it

Varsity sweaters always seem like they're sized for men. The baggy XXL look may have been all the rage paired with leggings when you were a student, but it was meant to be a temporary college cover-up. Remember, anything that doesn't give you a shape is bound for the recycle bin. Get that sweater out of your closet and cheer for another team.

best bets

Check out how a blast from the past can be done the right way, with class, while still taking you down memory lane at www.modcloth.com.

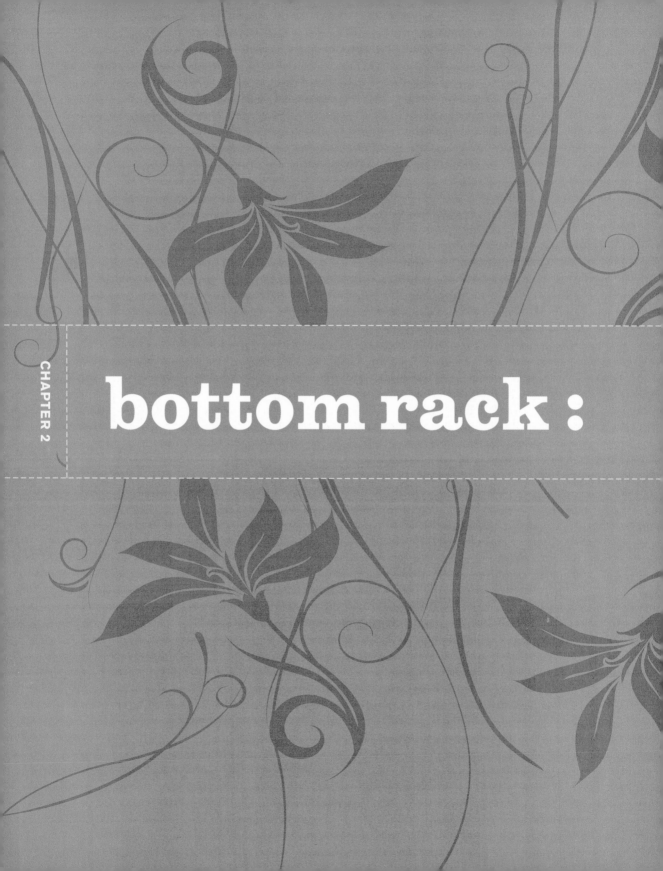

bottom rack :

pants & skirts

wear

Classic cut straight-leg trousers with center crease and medium waistband.

+ A pant with a fitted waistband that doesn't pinch or buckle

+ A rise (the measurement from crotch to button) that feels right; average rise is about ten inches, for jeans it's four to eight inches

+ A pant that gives you a nicely molded derrière

+ Fabrics that drape but have structure from waist to foot, such as cotton or wool blends, linen, cotton twill, and tweed

+ Denim that doesn't cut off your circulation

+ Nothing too tight (no pressing against your body) and nothing so loose that it chafes between your legs or creates folds

IT'S A STEAL

For designer pants at discount prices with easy-to-navigate visuals, try www.bluefly.com > shop categories > pants (then refine your search by price with a cool slide-and-click price bar). If you shop during seasonal sales, you can save up to 80 percent.

OUTSOURCING

Your pants hem should hit the middle of your heel, or a bit longer if you like length (do not go shorter). Find stores that offer free hemming with purchase, such as Banana Republic's Luxe customer rewards program.

SOLE MATES

A pointy or peep-toe pump or heeled sandal is the ultimate match for classic trousers. The thicker the heel, the heavier the feel: wear with wide-legged pants. Flats are best with cropped styles for a gamine-chic look.

SHAPE SAVER

How do you achieve no VPL (visible panty lines) if you *really* like your panties? Try the **save-me** Soma Intimates Vanishing Edge panties, which are soft, comfy and VPL-free. They're available in boyshort, brief, bikini, hipster, four for $36; www.soma.com, 866-768-7662.

- Elastic waistbands
- Buttons or clasps that barely hold your waistband together
- A tight waistband that dissects your body into two distinct halves
- A rise you can feel (too tight or too loose)
- Unflattering colors from another era (acid wash is fashionable only once in a blue moon)
- Overalls
- Cuffs that are wider than your ankles
- Jeans that bunch up at your ankles
- Pegged varieties (pants that taper with or without a closure or a tight roll at the cuff)
- Hems that drag on the floor

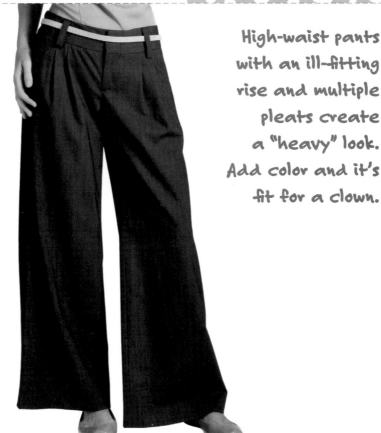

High-waist pants with an ill-fitting rise and multiple pleats create a "heavy" look. Add color and it's fit for a clown.

raising the bar
Have a tummy? Side pockets that pooch out are your enemies. Use my TV trick: Get Fashion-Fix—apparel and body tape by Topstick. Place the double-sided tape just inside pocket seams and flatten. This will streamline pockets for a day. It's $7.99; go to www.vapon.com for stores.

ditch it
There's no excuse for muffin-top spillage. You need a looser waistband or one that doesn't dip so low (which accents your body at the hips). Pants should fit all your curves: waist, hips, and thighs. Buy up a size and take in the waist, if necessary, for a better fit.

behind the seams
Cuffed pants generally shorten legs. Pleats almost always draw attention to undesirable places. Pockets can add visual pounds to hips.

sale suckers
A red flag for a bad rise is when you feel it. If it presses against you, it's too tight (and most likely too revealing). If you feel chafing between your thighs, your rise is riding too low.

wear

Streamlined drop-waist pants without embellishment or front-flap pockets.

other must HAVES

+ **Low-rise khakis**
+ **Low-rise jeans**
+ **Legging pants**

RAISING THE BAR

Proportion is key when balancing your torso with the right pants. If you are short-waisted, create the illusion of a longer torso with a low-waist pant that dips below your waist. If you are long-waisted, make legs leggier with a high-waist pant. Refrain from the extreme in either direction.

IT'S A STEAL

Gilt Groupe (www.gilt.com) is an invitation-only online sample sale that features different top designers and their wares each week. It often includes separates, like pants, at heavily discounted prices. Get a friend to sign up and receive a $25 credit toward your next purchase.

SHAPE SAVER

Just say no to butt cracks and belly buttons with JAKs—a stretch lace bandeau for your waist that supports your tum and covers any revealing flesh. Pull JAKS on over your pants until it overlaps with the edge of the waist. The result? You look like you have a sweet, layered camisole on under your shirt. Available in white, beige, and black from Miss Oops, $38; www.missoops.com.

SOLE MATES

As a short-waisted wonder myself, I tend to hem my low-rise pants barely above the ground and pair them with a high heel. This way, I salvage some leg length while the low waist makes my torso look longer.

waist watchers!

Where your hands rest on your torso is your natural waistline. An inch or more below the natural waistline is considered low-rise and an inch or more above, high-rise.

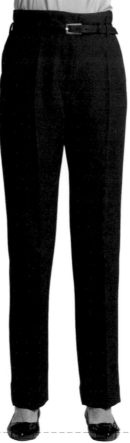

Ultra high-waist pant in a heavy fabric and a cut that thickens thighs and tightens across hips.

other must LOSE

- **High-waisted bell bottoms**
- **High-waisted harem pants**
- **High-waisted gauchos**—only for those who know how to wear them (with boots!)

raising the bar

When *do* you get to wear wide-leg pants? As with all separates, think proportionally. If you are thin, then wear slim-cut pants. If you are plus-size, wear a wider width pant to bring balance to your upper half.

age alert

For a long time, high-waisted pants were a style staple. For many women, it's a tough cut to give up because of a *sense* of added support around the stomach. But ironically, if you sport a stomach, a heavy bottom, or a short upper torso, high-waisted pants cut off your proportions in the worst way. Don't age yourself even more by wearing pants from a past era.

best bets

For those who are long-waisted and need quality high-waist pants, don't fear: Jones New York specializes in luxe crepe pants with stretch (about $100).

match point

When so many things can go wrong with this pant, make your top right. Wear it tucked or cropped.

sale suckers

As a petite woman the best high-waist pant is one with a slimmer cut. While the high waist is meant to give you a longer leg, a wide, generous cuff will make you look like a squashed sailor.

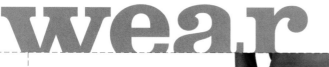

wear

Flat-front, pleated pants, with a tapered hem in a fabric that conforms to your body shape.

other must HAVES

+ Belted, cropped **karate pants** that appear to wrap around the waist

+ Full-length pleated pants

RAISING THE BAR

Pleats worn well add dimension and shape to pants without adding unwanted weight to curves. Because they can lengthen legs (and who doesn't want that?), I say embrace this masculine trouser with a twist. As a starting point, limit yourself to one, two, or three flat pleats per pant panel.

MATCH POINT

Balance the volume that pleats create below the waist with a sleek top above. Tailored blouses and tanks work best. Tuck and belt if you can for a deliciously defined waist.

BEST BETS

I don't know a woman on the planet who doesn't pine for the perfect fitting black pants. Enter The Gap with Black Magic, a new premium collection of seven black pant styles that start at $49.50. Still troubled by a bad fit? They have experts on staff to help you work some *real* magic.

IT'S A STEAL

Before purchasing pants online, check for discount codes and free shipping codes at www.retailmenot.com and www.freeshipping.org.

ever wonder where the name for capris came from?

Created in 1948, capri pants are named after the Italian isle of Capri by designer Sonja de Lennart.

M.C. Hammer-era harem pants in an exaggerated cut with a deeply dropped crotch, heavily gathered waist, and a tapered hem.

other must LOSE

- Ankle bow-tie, **pegged harem pants**
- **Baggy pants**

ditch it

Harem pants almost never come back into vogue. Meant for the super skinny and tall, they rarely have redeeming qualities for the rest of us with hips and thighs and tummies.

behind the seams

The style of pleat is crucial to how it will lie. Knife pleats—perhaps the most common found on pants and skirts—are best when spaced apart and not gathered one atop the other. Box pleats—two back-to-back knife pleats—are common on skirts (think plaid school uniforms) and can add bulk to the stomach if spaced close together.

sale suckers

Pleats that extend over the hips and super loose pleats that run the length of the leg can make hips and thighs look twice as big. Harem pants with pegged legs generally make the hips look doubly wide, like an inverted triangle.

wear

A cropped straight-leg, flat-front pant that ends at mid-calf or slightly below, with flat pockets and no pleats in a versatile, neutral color.

other must HAVES

+ Belted **khaki capris** for a great, crisp look

+ **Just below-the-knee capris** for those who love their calves

+ **Capris with side slits** for a slightly sexy alternative

RAISING THE BAR

A thick belt will make a capri pant top-heavy. Consider a skinny or thin (one-inch) belt instead. Against a solid color like navy or tan, a metallic belt adds shine and modernizes the look. Swap out a formal belt for a casual, colorful scarf only if you want to zero in attention on your hips.

SHAPE SAVER

Feel like skipping panties? Go commando in Commandos organic cotton patches that adhere directly to jeans or pants, eliminating visible panty lines while providing cotton comfort. Eight patches are $18; www.gocommandos.com.

MATCH POINT

The easiest top to wear with capris is one that ends at or a little below the waistband. Beware if your babydoll or jersey top ends at the hips; it will make them look wider than a shopping cart!

SOLE MATES

Feminine flats perfectly complete capris, whether we're talking cute jeweled styles, sandals with rosettes or flowers, or closed-toe with cutouts or bows. Unless you want to appear super tall, skip the sky-high skinny heels. A medium (two-inch) to lower heel is an all-around safer bet, and the wider the better to match a capri's casual cut.

AGE ALERT

If you have thick ankles, big feet, or heavy lower calves, capri pants will highlight these areas, so avoid them no matter your age.

Wrinkled, baggy cargo pants with patch pockets and sloppily tied drawstrings at the waist and leg openings.

other must LOSE

- Untapered, military-style **camouflage pants**

- **Utility pants** overflowing with pockets and ties

- **Loose jumpsuit pants**

ditch it

Cargos with more pockets than you can count create added baggage on your body: read "pouchy kangaroo." Pockets placed on hips and thighs make everything fatter. Ignore the pocket's stashing ability and save your knickknacks for your purse.

age alert

As we age, the tendency is to go for a roomier, wider pant leg to balance a growing tummy, hips, or both. But a baggy cargo can be too extreme.

Embrace a cargo with a simplified silhouette (only a few pockets) and as slim a cut as your frame can handle—one that graces your thighs without creasing when you sit.

outsourcing

Don't try to "make" cropped pants yourself. I'm talking to those women out there who roll their pants all the way up to their knees or who hack at them with scissors to make cut-offs. Take them to a tailor, where the professional snip and sew will cost you all of $10.

shining moment

The cargo's casual street style doesn't lend itself to delicate jewelry like wispy necklaces, lacy earrings, or skinny bracelets. Go for a bold cuff or a statement-making watch, like a Timex women's leather-banded chronograph watch.

temperature rising

Some sport cargos zipper off at the knee to offer a cool alternative. Hand-rolled cuffs can add visual chunkiness to calves—not very cool at all, huh?

wear

Fitted, boot-cut jeans in a dark denim wash that nicely frames your booty and legs, paired with high heels.

other must HAVES

+ **Trouser denim pants**, perfect for a casual or artistic workplace environment

+ **Skinny jeans** for under fuller sweaters and blousy tops

+ **Cropped denim** for warmer months

+ **Jeggings** (jean leggings)

RAISING THE BAR

Enter your measurements and style preferences at www.mytruefit.com, and find jean options across brands that best match your body. Experts suggest looking for jeans with at least 2 percent stretch.

SHAPE SAVER

Like to wear your denim with heels *and* flats? Bristols 6 Hem Tape for Denim is super sticky **save-me** double-stick tape, allowing you to give jeans a temporary hem for whichever shoe you choose ($12, bristols6.com).

BEST BETS

Cookie Johnson (Magic Johnson's wife) was sick of not getting jeans on past her knees. Her denim line, CJ by Cookie Johnson, offers jean cuts with curvy women in mind: stretch, dark washes, and higher rise in rear. Nordstrom, $141 and up; www.nordstrom.com/cjcookiejohnson.com.

SHAPE SAVER

Have a pancake butt? Look for back pockets placed high on your rear to give you an instant derrière lift and curve. And keep the pockets clean.

MATCH POINT

Wide-legged, dark denim trousers are fast becoming office staples and a **save-me** for women who love wearing jeans to work. Isaac Mizrahi for Liz Claiborne and Nicole by Nicole Miller offer stunning options.

toss

Oversized, formless denim that is cut too short, in a high rise and a light wash that doesn't flatter thighs.

other must LOSE

- **Stovepipe jeans** if you have curves
- **Acid wash jeans**
- **Super tight jeans** that create butt wrinkles under cheeks—too tight!

behind the seams
Distressed, stonewashed, faded, and whiskered jeans (all techniques to make the jeans look worn) can make legs wider when the special effects are positioned at the hips and thighs. If these are problem areas, opt for darker washes with consistent color. I size up when it comes to darker denim beause darker jeans have less stretch.

outsourcing
Going up a jean size to fit your thighs and butt commonly results in the drafty "back gap" at the waist that no amount of belting can correct. Have a tailor do the easy work of taking in the waist.

age alert
"How low can you go" is not a motto for low-rise jeans as you mature. While still flaunting your assets, make sure jeans fully cover your butt, lower back, and tummy. Brands such as Paige Premium Denim and 7 For All Mankind offer ample options.

insourcing
Did you know that jeans fade with every wash? To preserve pigment, turn jeans inside out before washing in cold water. Check the label to see if tumble dry on low heat is recommended; otherwise, hang dry.

ditch it
Tapered denim shows off calves and legs but also makes hips appear twice as wide. Very few can wear skinny stovepipe jeans (which are cut narrow from knee to ankle). Save this style for boyish figures with no hips.

37

jeans for real women

Since the rise of designer jeans in the 1970s, there is now more figure-flattering denim available than ever before. Here's a breakdown of the major players in the jeans world and the best cuts they offer.

the brand	the style	tips & where to buy
CITIZENS OF HUMANITY	KELLY Bootcut—slick denim AVA Straight-leg—*Access Hollywood* voted this the best straight-leg jean in 2009 AVEDON Super Stretch Skinny; Avedon Slick Skinny Leg and the Stirrup Skinny Leg—uses their exclusive 818 Super Stretch denim with 35 percent stretchability, standard five-pocket. It's a jean that wears like a legging and is super soft; 8-inch front rise, 30-inch inseam, 11-inch leg opening. Also available in a stirrup.	Creative director Jerome Dahan sews side seams at an angle, not straight, for a slimming effect. Available at www.citizensofhumanity.com
CJ BY COOKIE JOHNSON	Debuted with five styles, all with generous rises. Three examples: FAITH (straight-leg) 9-inch rise, 34-inch inseam, 14-inch leg opening TRUTH (high-waist, wide-leg) 10.5-inch rise, 24-inch leg opening, 34.5-inch inseam GLORY (pleated jean) 9.25-inch rise, 13-inch leg opening, 23.5-inch inseam	Available at Nordstrom, Neiman Marcus, and Bloomingdales, http://cjbycookiejohnson.com
GAP	1969 CURVY JEANS with boot-cut leg opening—offer a little extra room in the hips, thighs, and seat with a "contoured waistband" that sucks in the hips. Choose ankle, regular, or long inseam.	Available at www.gap.com
HUDSON	CANONBURY Five-Pocket Bootcut—double-button waistband and classic boot-cut fit. 19-inch leg opening, 34½-inch inseam	Available at www.hudsonjeans.com
J BRAND	SCARLETT Curvy Fit Bootcut—fuller in the thigh and high hip, with a contoured waistband that eliminates any waist gap so many women with curves encounter. 18-inch leg opening, 34-inch inseam, 12.5-ounce stretch denim	J Brand is known for a slimmer fit in the leg, dark washes, clean back pockets and jeans without embellishments. Available at www.jbrandjeans.com
JOE'S JEANS	THE HONEY—famous for its fit on voluptuous women. The waistband is "clinched" or cinched in the rear to fit curvy women in the thighs and hips, and particularly their bottoms, so no back gap. 18¾-inch leg opening THE SKINNY HONEY—12½-inch leg opening THE MUSE—high waist that lands just below the belly button to hold in the tummy. A "lower than usual high waist" and subtle pockets to "stop any undesirable extra curves that many high-waist fits present." Boot-cut leg with 19-inch leg opening, 34-inch inseam, 9-inch rise.	Available at www.joesjeans.com

LEVI STRAUSS & CO.	TOTALLY SLIMMING Boot-cut Jeans—these best-sellers, made with high-stretch denim, feature a built-in tummy control panel for an ultimate slim look. TOTALLY SHAPING Jeans—feature high-stretch denim and built-in tummy control panel, with a backside engineered to flatter the booty.	Available at Kmart (www.kmart.com), Wal-mart (www.walmart.com), and www.levi.com
LUCKY BRAND	RILEY SLOUCHY SKINNY Jeans—a cross between a boyfriend jean and a skinny jean that Lucky Brand dubs the "liberated skinny." Flatters the curvier figure because of the rise, pocket placement, and general silhouette, with a relaxed fit through the hips and thighs. 32-inch regular inseam	Available at www.luckybrand.com
PAIGE PREMIUM DENIM	MONTECITO—generous in the thighs and derrière, a tailored boot cut that still achieves a slim leg. 8-inch rise, 34-inch inseam, 18-inch leg opening HIDDEN HILLS Carbon High-Rise Bootcut—a higher rise and a double-button waistband add support in the waist. 9-inch rise, 34-inch inseam, 20-inch leg opening	Available at www.paigepremiumdenim.com and www.paigeusa.com
7 FOR ALL MANKIND	JOSEPHINA Skinny Boyfriend Jeans—slightly roomy in the thigh but tapered in the leg. 7-inch front rise, 11.5-inch back rise, 11.5-ounce stretch Italian denim, 2 percent spandex GINGER PANT in lightweight Mercer—this brand's widest trouser skims over thighs to a wide leg opening. 8-inch front rise, 12-inch back rise	Available at www.7forallmankind.com
SERFONTAINE	SWEETHEART JEANS—a popular, classic style with special stretch fabric and a curved yoke (waistband) on the backside to flatter derrières. Strategically placed pockets do double duty: flatter curvy bottoms and give the illusion of curves for the straighter woman. Serfontaine uses a patented bio-stretch technology (a four-way stretch fabric) so the styles are exceptionally flattering no matter what your body type. Available in Sweetheart boot-cut legs (7.5-inch front rise, 16-inch leg opening) and drainpipe legs (straight but not skinny; 7.5-inch front rise and 13-inch leg opening).	In U.S. stores, the Serfontaine body-scanning machine enables shoppers to have their bodies scanned and get jeans and size recommendations that best fit their specific body types; custom-made jeans can be ordered based on the scans. For stores, www.serfontaine.com
TRUE RELIGION	BECKY Boot-cut Jeans—one of True Religion's core cuts, comes in a variety of styles, embellishments, and washes. 8-inch front rise, 13-inch back rise, 18-inch leg opening	Available at www.truereligionbrandjeans.com

A former model turned founder of an eponymous line of premium denim, Paige Adams-Geller has blazed a path for women to find their perfect pair of jeans. After years of working as a design consultant and building a reputation as a "fit doctor" for Guess jeans, 7 For All Mankind, True Religion, and other companies, she channeled her knowledge into her own line, Paige Premium Denim, which offers a broad range of silhouettes for every body type. With down-to-earth sass, she reveals mistakes to avoid, styling to embrace, and the only reason you may arm yourself with scissors, and take denim matters into your own hands.

Paige Premium Denim is synonymous with fit. Can you speak about the range of your specialty denim?

I offer many different silhouettes and rises so that a woman can find her perfect pair. We use the finest quality denim that keeps its shape, and hours are spent on fit so that your butt looks perky, your legs look long and lean, and your hips look smaller. Every girl's dream, right?

What are the faux pas you hate to see when it comes to jeans?

Say no to crack! There is nothing attractive about butt cleavage. It is never, under any circumstance, flattering to see underwear of any kind sticking out of the top of your jeans. It's just not classy! When trying on jeans, do the sit-down test in the dressing room. If you see crack, try on a pair with a slightly higher back rise. We will all thank you for it.

Another major pet peeve is the muffin top. You can wear jeans that are sexy that also control the side spillage. A good mid-rise or high-rise style in a slim fit will give you the look you want minus the spillover that, well…nobody wants. Find a pair where the waistband hits right at the spillage spot. The waistband acts as a control top, holding the side spills and giving you a smooth shape and a sexy look.

Let's talk about length and shoes.

Crops are cute, but floods are not. Jeans should not drag the floor when wearing high heels, but they should not be more than an inch above the heel either. I know this poses a problem when you want a jean that is versatile, but for fashion's sake, decide if the jean you have is more of a flats or a heels jean and get it hemmed accordingly.

What's the best directive to give a tailor?

Ask him to keep the "original hem" to retain the integrity of the design. The tailor will actually shorten the jean and re-attach the original hem.

Any pet peeves with how people wear denim?

I'm not a fan of denim jackets worn with denim jeans of the same color. Denim should not be worn as a jumpsuit. Try wearing a white or black denim vest or jacket with your blue jeans, or throw on an indigo denim vest or jacket with your black, gray, or white jeans. My favorite look is a leather jacket with a T-shirt or tank and jeans. Also ladies, please, no cropped jeans with Crocs for anything other than gardening. Try a cute pair of gladiator sandals or ballet flats. Much more chic and just as comfortable!

What are some of the latest technologies with jeans that are bringing comfort and fit to denim and to women of all sizes?

There are so many technological advancements in fabrics and fibers. Super stretch fabric in denim is a huge part of the current and upcoming collections. What makes a fabric super stretch is a 360-degree stretchability and a much higher concentration of stretch than traditional denim. Super stretch denims hug the body, holding you in while providing the ultimate comfort. An important super stretch fiber is the T400. It's chlorine-resistant and can withstand bleaching and washing techniques not typically used on stretch denim. The latest treatments, such as antique finishes, whisker washing, and sand blasting, can be applied to garments with excellent results. Garments not only fit well, but retain their shape wear after wear. Super stretches are perfect for the legging and jegging (a hybrid of tight jeans and leggings) trends in lighter weight denims. Heavier weight super stretches will become important in the fall and winter seasons for more traditional cuts.

With your vast expertise on this topic, any secret style-saving tips when it comes to wearing jeans and figure flattery?

If you're shorter-waisted or petite, a lower rise will give you a more proportioned fit, whereas someone with a longer torso might want to opt for a higher rise jean to get that same proportioned look. There are also five different body types that I like to think of as jewels rather than fruits! To find your body type and the perfect fit for you, go to www.paigeusa.com and answer the questions on my fit guide. I will personally help you!

Will you share some practical shopping advice to help us find the right pair of jeans?

Shopping for denim is as tedious and uncomfortable as shopping for swimsuits, so keep in mind your assets. What do you like about your body? What do you want to find in a jean to make you feel and look your best? I also like to make sure I have the kind of shoes and top with me that I would likely wear with those jeans, to try on in the dressing room so I can make sure that I will be happy with the overall look.

Any parting words for the perfect fit seekers?

Last but not least, *ignore the size label!* Don't get frustrated over the number on a tag. I cannot stress this enough. There is no standard in sizing, so it really means nothing. Some brands follow a more European style sizing, some follow a more American style sizing, which makes it very confusing for the consumer. I always say grab what you think your size is and then grab a size below that and above that and try them all on.

So ditch the tag!

The fit is what makes you feel and look great, not the digits on the inside of the jean. Nobody but you even sees that. And if it still bothers you, cut the tag out! After a few months, you won't even remember what size you bought. You'll only know how great you look and feel in your favorite pair of jeans.

bottom rack : pants

An A-line skirt in a neutral color and a flexible fabric that gently hugs hips, lies flat at the seams and falls nicely when paired with high heels.

+ A skirt that ends at your legs' most flattering point: where it makes your thighs, knees, or calves look their thinnest

+ An even hem that doesn't rise in the front, sides, or rear

+ A universally flattering style like the A-line skirt—no higher than knee-length but can go as low as the floor—and drapes flatteringly over hips and thighs

+ Unclingy fabrics

+ A zipper or buttons placed on your most slimming side

+ Flat pockets

+ A slit that doesn't gape when you move

+ A mid-length skirt long enough to cover the top of a boot

BEST BETS

Can't attend sample sales because you don't live in a major city? Still want to save up to 70 percent off retail for super-hip skirts? Enter Gilt Fuse (www.giltfuse.com), which offers online 36-hour sample sales on contemporary designs from Generra, Tracey Reese, French Connection, BCBG, and more. A sister site to Gilt Groupe, it's more "downtown" in style than the original. Not a member? E-mail membership@gilt.com.

RAISING THE BAR

A lesson on proportion: If your skirt is slim fitting, opt for a fuller blouse; a flared or fuller skirt demands a more tailored top. If you have a tummy, wear a dark color top that fits over the skirt's waistband.

SOLE MATES

The A-line skirt works with a ton of different shoe styles, from a pointy toe to a slight pump—even boots.

SHAPE SAVER

From the maker of the famed Bra-llelujah and footless pantyhose, Spanx has a new line of exquisite shapewear that helps you slim down while getting your sexy on. For skirts, try the Luscious Lace Mid-Thigh Shaper or the Sexy Sheer Mid-Thigh Shaper, $128 each; www.spanx.com.

- Skirts that crease at the hip fold, creating all-day wrinkles
- A style so tight you cannot easily sit or walk
- Dense pleats if you're hippy
- All around ruffles that create too much poof
- Fabrics that pull tightly (spandex) or pucker (seersucker) across the hips
- Denim styles that are too stiff
- Unflattering lengths that are too short or too long
- A poorly fitting cut that causes the waistband to ride up
- Horizontal panels of competing prints
- Shiny fabrics or sequins that make you look bottom-heavy
- Skirts that curve to your rear, creating "butt hump"

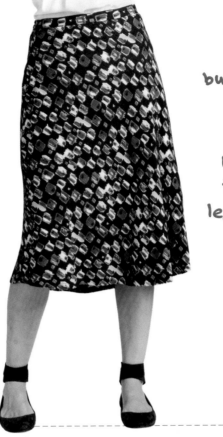

A three-quarter-length skirt in a busy print that hits at the thickest part of the calf, paired with shoes that compete for leg space, creating a stumpy look.

ditch it

Here's the deal: Three-quarter-length skirts land at the thickest part of the calves, which most of us want to hide, not highlight. Plus, they make legs look short. It's better to keep your hem either at your knees or at your feet rather than suspend it in the no-man's-land of middle calf-dom.

sole mates

Just when does a three-quarter-length skirt look more dynamite than drab? If you 1) have shapely calves; 2) can wear a slim-fitting boot that makes calves and ankles look trim; 3) already have long legs and don't need any additional lengthening below. For those who can handle it, pair this skirt with a fun mid-to-high heel or T strap—just no flats.

match point

A couple quick tips can save a three-quarter-length skirt and bring out its redeeming qualities. Pair it with a fitted top like a shapely sweater or a simple shirt that extends just beyond the waistline, and avoid bulky, shapeless tops or anything unbuttoned.

wear

An embellishment-free pencil skirt in a medium-weight fabric that lands at or slightly above the knee (within two inches) and is tapered at the hem.

other must HAVES

+ **Unexpected details** like rear exposed zippers or asymmetrical side buckles
+ **Slightly flared skirts**
+ **Skirts with single pleats** in front or back to draw attention to the legs
+ **Draped skirts**

BEST BETS
A pencil skirt is universally flattering—except for gals with thighs. Its straight up-and-down cut can balance out curves and taper to a sleek finish at or slightly above the knee, offering the slimmest of skirt fits. Bisou Bisou for JCPenney makes a small but impressive collection of beautifully tailored pencil skirts (www.jcp.com).

SOLE MATES
Flats ruin the length that a pencil skirt creates, so continue to flatter legs and feet with shoes that have a slight (one and a half inches) to tall (sky's the limit) heel.

AGE ALERT
If you've got gams, there isn't a sexier, more age-appropriate skirt to show some skin. Just don't go too long with this style, as it will age you. Likewise, a thick, heavy, long-sleeved shirt paired with a pencil skirt is a ticket straight to nowhere: It will make you look dowdy.

A full, short bell skirt that is gathered and pleated at the waistline like a bunched-up curtain, in a stiff fabric that adds even more bulk.

other must LOSE

- For someone with hips, a **super bell-shaped skirt or ultra-trim pencil skirt**

- **Bias-cut skirts** (cut on the diagonal) that cling to hips, unless you have a tiny bottom half

- **Wide-print plaid skirts** that draw attention to hips and thighs

- **Dirndl skirts** (a full skirt with gathers)

ditch it

Bell-shaped skirts (defined by a full skirt and a flared hem) are tough for anyone to wear because of the amount of volume they present. These gathered-at-the-waist skirts tend to enlarge the appearance of hips and waist.

match point

A poofy top plus a poofy skirt equals a marshmallow shape. Opt for a slim, tucked-in blouse for your own sweet perfection.

85 percent of all brand purchases are made by women

age alert

The fullness of a bell skirt is very playful and can turn heads when paired with shapely legs. It may even remind you of the youthfulness of cheerleaders. Yet, a sleeker silhouette is safer and more elegant as you age. Try a tailored full-length or pencil skirt instead.

A modern graphic print mini skirt with flat pockets and strappy shoes that complement the hues of the pattern.

other must HAVES

+ **Lace skirts** that offer visual texture but lie flat

+ **Sequined skirts**

+ **Drop-waist ruffled floral skirts**

SHAPE SAVER

Proportion is key to all your fashion choices, and the same goes for prints. If you have a big frame, go for big prints. If you're petite, smaller prints work for you. If in doubt, go with a mid-size print (say two inches square or larger) woven evenly throughout a fabric to hide imperfections that may lie underneath: protruding tummy, saddlebags, bumpy butt.

BEST BETS

For retro or ethnic-printed floral skirts, visit www.anthropologie .com. For vintage designer skirts (with a limited but ever-revolving selection) at enticing prices given the pristine quality, check out www.relicny.com.

BEHIND THE SEAMS

Trompe l'oeil fabrics make a skirt *look* like it's heavily embroidered when in fact it is a lightweight, woven masterpiece—thus its moniker, which means "trick of the eye."

49 percentage of women who find shapewear uncomfortable and thus don't wear it often

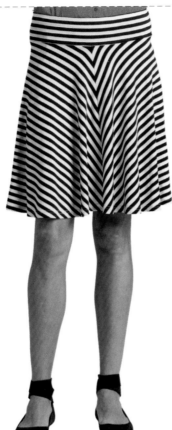

A dizzying striped skirt that adds poundage to the waist, in a thin, swinging fabric.

other must LOSE

- **Tiny prairie floral prints—** too casual for the workplace
- **Paisley prints**
- **Heavy knitted skirts**

sale suckers

If vertical stripes create length, horizontal stripes create width. If you have a midriff that bulges, a horizontal striped skirt will make an ample waist and hips appear even broader.

best bets

The starkness of a white stripe draws all eyes downward toward your lower half. Unless you're wearing a vertical pinstripe or a dark, wide-banded horizontal stripe à la Marc Jacobs, keep stripes and skirts separate.

match point

Stripes are an all-encompassing style statement, not to be mixed with other patterns—except for the truly fashion-forward few. But if you want to branch out from the obvious (pairing stripes with complementary solids), then here's how to mix your prints. Have a base color, the same color that is in all of your pieces. Pair one big print (like a graphic floral) with a smaller print (thin stripes). Introduce a third print when you get the hang of it.

wear

A slightly hip-hugging mini (eight inches above the knee) with interesting detail like bands or front ties, worn with tights.

other must HAVES

+ Perfect **short denim skirts**
+ **Khaki, cotton, or linen minis** for hotter months
+ **A-line minis in a heavier fabric** for work

SOLE MATES

I'm awestruck by catwalk models (and the models in this book) who can rock a mini in sky-high heels, but for the rest of womankind slipping across the kitchen floor, pair a mini with a little heel. Test on said kitchen floor for safety.

OUTSOURCING

No one wants a see-through skirt, but how to find a slip for a mini? Take the skirt to a tailor and plunk down about $25 to get a lining sewn in.

MATCH POINT

Nothing screams "styling pro" more than a neutral-hue mini skirt paired with textured or printed tights. Be hotter than hot and create shapely come-hither legs at the same time, as many tights now sport visually slimming designs like stripes or two-tone. Try www.wolford.com; Spanx's Tight-End Tights, which include shapewear for **save-me** style with compression (www.spanx.com); and Target's affordable Xhilaration tights.

ever wonder who made the miniskirt hip?

The founder of the Mod Look, British designer Mary Quant, is largely credited for its creation in the 1950s, giving it a name and a major following.

A super short micro mini skirt (higher than eight inches!), with the pocket lining visible through holes or below the hem.

other must LOSE

- **Revealing micro minis** that show anything anatomical other than the leg

- **Clingy spandex minis**

- **See-through micro-mini skirts**

raising the bar

Don't get me wrong. I love a super short skirt and even have a few in which my husband warns me not to bend over. But micro minis are for the chosen few of super gam-dom. If you wear one, know that your legs are open to complete public gawking…and scrutiny.

ditch it

If you're asking yourself, "Is this too short?" you've answered your own question.

age alert

Although I don't like rules when it comes to age and skirts, if you want a guideline, keep it at the knee. From there, try going a little shorter, until your inner wisdom says it's high enough.

temperature falling

Live in a cold clime and find mini skirts too drafty? With truly rockin' thick tights, leggings, and the most stylish of knee-high or above-the-knee boots available, there's no longer a reason to write off a short length (try www.hue.com).

wear

A long skirt in a mid-weight fabric that flows around the hips and waist, with a fun touch like a ruffled hem paired with statement-making flats.

other must HAVES

+ **Long A-line skirts**
+ **Tiered Boho skirts** with length
+ **Elegant** evening, floor-length **skirt separates**
+ **Boho skirts with one print or complementary prints**

OUTSOURCING

Always wanted to be tall? A long skirt can add height and conceal a myriad of leg imperfections through its long, uninterrupted column of color and fabric. A long skirt should *appear* to nearly touch the floor. Put on your shoes before you have it hemmed to skim just above.

BEST BETS

Wish you had a fairy godmother to whip you up that special occasion dress for one night? Enter www.renttherunway.com, where you can rent a designer (Badgley Mischka, Prabal Gurung, and Robert Rodriguez to name a few) dress and jewelry for 4-8 days at 10% of the actual cost. For the return, slip your rentals into a pre-paid package and mail: the company handles the dry cleaning. Terrified about fit? You get to choose two sizes of the same dress. Bippity boppity boo!

SOLE MATES

I'm sick of seeing Olive Oyl thick platforms with super long skirts. The look is clunky and chunky, and more punky than professional; it ruins the intended length of a long skirt with stubby feet. Yes, your soles should get more substantial the longer your hemline, but that means a slightly thicker heel—not a stage. Believe it or not, flats are fabulous for this look because the skirt does all the lengthening you need.

A long, drapey skirt that is billowy and Bohemian, with a wide, elastic waistband and competing prints.

other must LOSE

- **Long, stiff cargo skirts** with drawstring tie
- **Long wrap-around skirts** that easily flap open
- **Heavily embroidered long skirts**

it's a steal

Sign up for Ebates, a cash-back shopping web site, and get an average of 2 to 10 percent cash back. Just go to www.ebates .com and choose from 1200 retailers you want to make a purchase from. Ebates will then redirect you to the store's web site and, if you buy something there, credit you with a percentage of cash back. The list of participating stores is impressive, and includes Saks Fifth Avenue (2.5 percent back), Kate Spade (3.5 percent), Macy's (5 percent), and Max Studio (6 percent).

sale suckers

Don't forget that a skirt's shape has the power to flatter—or shatter—your figure. Bell, full, trumpet, and flare skirts can add roundness to your bottom half, while pencil, A-line, and slim-fit minis offer a sleeker silhouette. (See pages 52-53 for more on skirt hems.)

22 percentage of women who shop online at least once a day

51

skirting the issue

Ever wonder about the names of all those skirts and how best to wear them? Below is an inventory of ten popular skirts, identified by hem. I've included my tip-top styling tips so you can wear them with confidence.

skirt hem	defined		tip-top styling tips
BANDED	This is characterized by bands of fabric wrapping around the skirt, like a bandage.		Shockingly flattering because it sucks you in, the banded skirt can deceptively function like shapewear despite its clinginess, even for those with hips and a tummy. A-line skirts that use bands as accents are the comfortable alternative.
EYELET	Eyelet embroidery is a technique that punches holes in fabric to create lace-like patterns.		Since eyelet is so often made with cottons and linens, it's synonymous with spring/summer and light, breezy looks. Keep your top casual and avoid eyelet on eyelet—too busy to the eye.
PETAL/TULIP	Fabric is layered to drape like overlapping flower petals. (Picture the shape of an upside-down tulip.)		When short, this style can increase volume around the hips. The longer the hem, the more weighted the fabric and the slimmer the silhouette. Pair with a tucked-in blouse.
SCALLOPED	Like a scallop shell, this skirt sports a series of rounded curves.		Knee-length or shorter is the ideal for this skirt, as the scalloping adds weight. Pair with dainty shoes to match the femininity of this look.
TRUMPET	A straight skirt that flares at the hem.		This skirt is for the hipless; otherwise you might look like a mermaid. The trumpet is best between knee-length and three-quarter-length. Save floor-length for formal event wear, like a wedding gown.

skirt hem	defined	tip-top styling tips
LACE/ RUFFLED	Lace comprises the entire skirt, or panels, or the hem of the skirt and is usually lined; Ruffled is tiers of fabric.	For black lace, avoid light-color underlays, which widen and negatively enhance your silhouette; A full ruffled skirt is not for everybody, particularly those with full hips and thighs.
BUBBLE	This skirt is defined by hems that are sewn and tucked under to create a ballooning poof.	The bubble skirt can hide wide thighs and add spunk to your everyday attire. The key is a wide waistband to slim the waist. Pair with tights and heels.
CAST SHADOW/ OVERLAY	One layer of longer fabric, (can be gossamer, like tulle) overlays another layer of solid fabric (or vice versa) revealing itself at the hem.	This style complements many body types and can be worn with appeal at a variety of lengths. This is a dressier hem, so pair with more formal footwear like heels.
LASER CUT	A laser is used to cut the fabric of this skirt and/ or hem. The laser cut design can range from individual petals to lace-like cutouts.	Because laser cutting can be intricate, keep shoes simple: solid colors, clean styles—nothing with too many cutouts or straps.
UNFINISHED	Often associated with cutoff jean skirts, an unfinished hem looks like the seamstress didn't complete the work: dangling threads, uneven cut, jagged finish.	The unfussiness of the unfinished hemline gives off a casual vibe, so embrace flats, shorter heels, or boots.

SKIRT HEMS

bottom rack : skirts

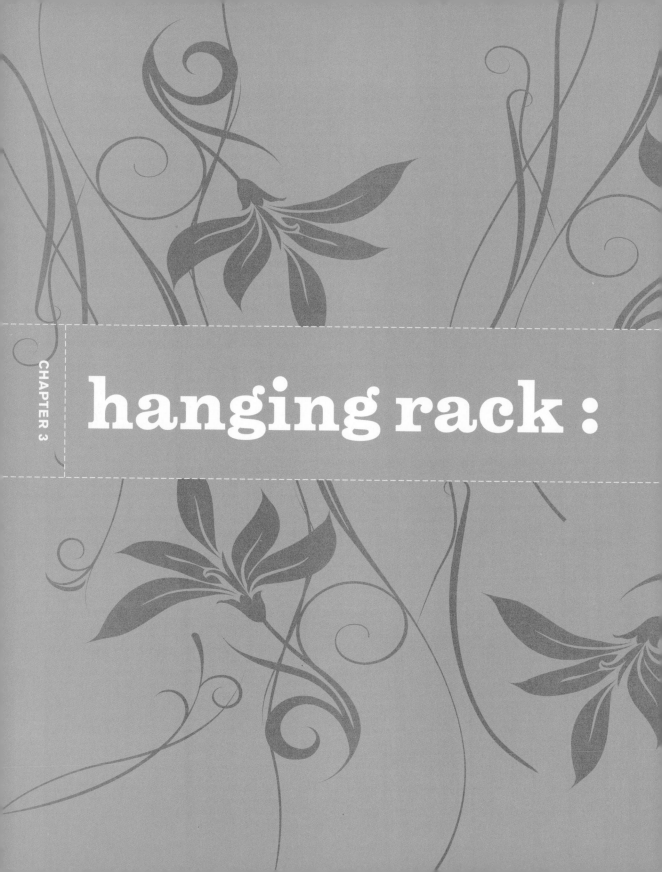

hanging rack :

dresses, suits & coats

wear

A V-neck, semi-fitted dress, worn with a bold necklace or statement earrings, a bracelet, and heels.

+ Shoulder straps or fabric that rests naturally on your shoulders

+ Armholes that fit— no gaping, no constricting

+ A zipper that zips easily. Holding your breath? Size up

+ Seams that lie flat on shoulders, sides, and butt

+ A style that tastefully shows some skin in your décolleté to balance a curvy body

+ Fabric that drapes smoothly, showing off curves without being taut

+ Monochrome color scheme, which is almost always slimming

+ Patterns proportional to your body size. If you're petite, go for smaller prints; for larger frames, try bigger prints

IT'S A STEAL

For the best prices on designer dresses, turn to www.theoutnet.com. Founded by the creators of www.Net-A-Porter.com and launched in spring 2009, this exclusive online outlet offers top designers at deeply discounted prices (how about 3.1 Phillip Lim, Fendi, or Givenchy at 80 percent off?!).

SHINING MOMENT

Pairing jewelry with dresses is all about the neckline. General tips: For a square, scoop, sweetheart, or structured neckline, wear earrings and a bracelet. For a high neckline, strapless, or V-neck, wear a statement-making necklace. For the strapless, the necklace may be above or below the neckline, while for the V-neck, generally stay within the V for no overlap.

INSOURCING

A dress wrinkles only where you sit in it. Rather than dry cleaning or professionally pressing after one wear, spray on Wrinkle Free Clothing Fabric Spray ($5.50 for three ounces; www.amazon.com) to smooth out wrinkles in ten seconds.

- Beyond busy prints
- Horizontal stripes (unless you're curve-less)
- Shoulder fabric or straps that dig
- Unflatteringly stiff fabrics
- Roomy, shapeless dresses that no longer fit
- A dress with sky-high shoulder pads
- Shirt dresses with buttons that pop at the chest
- Overly appliquéd styles with sequins, paillettes, rhinestones, rosettes, beading, crystals, pom poms, fringe, and shells that visually or actually weigh you down
- Strapless styles if you have broad shoulders
- Muu-muus

A visually detailed dress with busy pattern panels is never a basic choice.

BASIC DRESS

hanging rack : dresses

shining moment

Don't layer jewels on top of a printed dress, which already has enough visual attraction. Stick to simple earrings or a bangle and let the dress speak for itself.

age alert

Showing more skin as you age does not necessarily translate to sexy. An open décolleté and sleeveless dress work if your chest is smooth and clear and your arms are toned. Sport a slit if you love your legs, but if it's too high, your dress will blow away with a big gust of wind. Assess your assets, find your comfort zone, and leave plunging cuts for the red carpet.

shape saver

Spaghetti straps offer no reprieve if you're busty. Go for thicker straps (that are still thin enough to show off shoulders) and a great bra to match. Soma's new Custom Support Bra with its trademarked Smart Cup design promises the right support and lift based on cup size; all that breast support, plus straps that are actually *pretty* ($42; www.soma.com).

wear

A crisp, belted shirtdress in a monochromatic color scheme with short sleeves and plenty of charming details, like ruffled sleeves or a tie belt.

other must HAVES

+ **Tailored, nipped-at-the-waist sheaths**
+ **Wrap dresses**
+ **Long-sleeve shirtdresses**

RAISING THE BAR

The tailored, belted shirtdress flatters a wide range of silhouettes and is a standalone piece—you don't need a coat or other trimmings to dress it. If you want to punch it up, swap the original belt for one in a bright or contrasting color. For reasonable options, try www.mangoshop.com.

MATCH POINT

Most people equate "shirtdress" with going on safari, but think beyond Africa. Look for details like flap pockets, braided belts, flirty cap sleeves, and workplace-appropriate prints (keep it one color to best flatter). Match with pumps or flats, but don't overload accessories on this already structured look.

SHINING MOMENT

The open neckline most shirtdresses provide allows room for a statement necklace (pair with a bold bangle or stacked bracelets to personalize the look). For jewelry with a global vibe, try Stefani Greenfield's Curations on HSN. Greenfield, former co-owner of the chic Scoop boutiques, launched Curations in March 2009. Teardrop rings, floral cuffs, Aztec drop necklaces, and other jewelry start as low as $28 (www.hsn.com > fashion > curations).

A gossamer tunic dress that looks like a nightie and is too short in length and too big in volume.

other must LOSE

- **Drop-waist tunics** with ruffle hem

- **Tunics with an oversize chunky belt**: read frumpy

ditch it

Tunics are all the rage, but many styles do your body absolutely no favors. If the color washes you out, is too short or too see-through, no one will be looking at you; they'll be looking embarrassingly *through* you.

best bets

Ever wonder why you're a size 8 for one designer and a 12 for another? E Dressme New York and its sister site, www.edressme .com, finally decode sizing. Put your measurements in the "Find My Size" search feature and get your best size for specific designers. They also feature fun dress collections like "work dresses," "celebrity dresses," and "I love Paris." Famous designers include Tracy Reese, Twelfth Street by Cynthia Vincent, and Nanette Lepore. Free shipping on returns in the United States.

age alert

Why doesn't this tunic work even for young women? Its lack of shape, of course. Even a Weight Watchers alumna or gym fanatic will find herself lost in all this fabric.

sole mates

Never expect a pair of statement shoes to rescue an already bad ensemble. A metallic sandal, heeled or flat, is the best choice to accompany a plain tunic, as it keeps within the general color scheme and adds a little pizzazz to a dull piece.

59

wear

A classic A-line silhouette in a solid color with front-flattering inverted pleats, a tailored top, and a fitted waist.

other must HAVES

+ All-purpose **little black dresses**
+ Colorful **cocktail dresses**
+ **A-line** silhouette **wrap dresses**
+ **Strapless dresses**, as long as you have some boobs to hold it up

RAISING THE BAR

I'm a dress devotee. You throw it on and off you go, without worrying about what to wear on the bottom. One of my favorite styles is the A-line cut, which is a classic **save-me** because it instantly minimizes hips with its fitted bodice and flowing lower skirt that falls gracefully over hips. And if you're as straight as a ruler, it'll give you a softer outline.

IT'S A STEAL

An all-around fantastic source for stylish frocks under $100 is Miss Me; www.missme.com.

SOLE MATES

A-lines extend your legs and make them look sexy long. This is a line you want to preserve, so go as low as a kitten heel. But feel free to bump up heel height as high as you feel comfortable.

BEHIND THE SEAMS

If you don't have curves, choose A-lines in structured fabrics like cotton, linen, and denim for day and thicker satins for evening—they offer a fuller flare. If you're curvy, an A-line in a softer drape reduces the volume you don't want; look for mid-weight, blends, and other flowy fabrics.

BEST BETS

A premier destination for antiques and furnishings, 1stdibs.com, has now added vintage designer fashions to the mix. An inspirational site for browsing dresses from past decades, it represents some of the finest vintage stores in the country. You may just find that perfect Christian Dior circa 1960 A-line dress you've been searching for. For favorite coast-to-coast vintage stores, try California-centric Wasteland (www.wastelandclothing.com) and New York's Screaming Mimi's (www.screamingmimis.com).

A bias-cut gown in a tight, synthetic material that clings and further accentuates the stomach and hips.

other must LOSE

- Clingy **silk gowns**
- **Skin-tight jersey dresses**
- **Gossamer slip dresses** with not enough coverage
- **Silk tank dresses**

behind the seams

Bias-cut essentially means cut at an angle. This can refer to the grain of the fabric, the forty-five-degree angle at which the fabric was cut, and/or the cut of the garment itself. Although it takes more fabric to create this style, a bias-cut gown tends to look like less when worn, because it hugs the body.

ditch it

How many people look sensational in bias-cut gowns? *Very few.* It's one of the toughest, most unforgiving styles for all body types. Why? Because it grazes over curves and flat stomachs and often gets stuck, like taffy on teeth, on hips or thighs. Try on a few. If you cannot walk straight without the fabric tugging in the other direction, then it probably doesn't look good.

best bets

Bias-cuts that fit are the ultimate in feminine dressing. Masters who do this well include Rebecca Taylor, J. Crew, and Vera Wang. Go for a lined dress in a mid-weight silk for more flow.

shape saver

You'll need to rein in unsightly bumps for this style. Try a full-body slimmer with an open neckline (think bathing suit with ultra compression!) like Yummie Tummie Sweetie Slip Dress, $86; www.yummietummie.com.

wear

An empire-waist dress perfectly fitted at the narrowest part of the upper ribcage, in a solid, print, or two tone.

other must HAVES

+ **Strapless empire-waist dresses**
+ **Halter dresses**, unless you have narrow, sloping, or meaty shoulders
+ **Keyhole dresses**

SHAPE SAVER

Those with boobs who shout "No way!" to the empire are right. This is *not* your style and will make you look like a cupcake with four layers of frosting spilling off the top. Because this silhouette cinches right under the bustline (which for many is the narrowest part of the torso), it can be exceedingly flattering—*unless* you want to draw the eye away from the chest.

IT'S A STEAL

Convertible dresses are the style *du jour* for wear-it-your-way versatility. DKNY's convertible dress ($195) works as both a strapless empire sheath and a skirt. For true fashion mileage, try the Twist Wrap Dress ($230; www.dessy .com/wrap-dress/), available in thirteen colors with seven suggested ways to wear it.

BEST BETS

To make this style look contemporary rather than something that walked out of a Renaissance Fair, reduce the volume, avoid velvets and other heavy fabrics, pick patterns that are evenly dispersed (not just on the top or bottom), and follow the talents of Carmen Marc Valvo, Michael Kors, and Miu Miu.

wear

A figure-hugging, sleeveless sheath that accentuates curves and lands above the knee, in a bold color with eye-catching detailing.

other must HAVES

+ **Shift dresses**, which have the potential to make you look a size smaller

+ **Trapeze dresses**—as forgiving as the shift and even roomier with a severe A-line

style to go

Sheath vs. Shift: Don't get these two dress styles confused. A sheath does not have a defined waistline, but the cut is tailored and/or darted to silhouette the waist so that it has a slight built-in curve. A shift is cut straight up and down in one solid line of fabric. For both, don't go longer than one inch below the knee. This includes sleeveless and sleeved options.

RAISING THE BAR

This style—showcasing curves with darts and a tailored midriff—is guaranteed to up the temperature on your sexy thermostat. Its fitted silhouette pairs nicely with a blazer and heels for work or a shrug and strappy sandals for evening.

IT'S A STEAL

I live for sample sales. One that brings many designers under one roof in cosmopolitan cities throughout the United States is Billion Dollar Babes. Up and operating since 2001, this "fashion club" attracts shoppers with seriously slashed prices. Can't make it to a sale? Try www.billiondollarbabes.com for six or more online sample sales a week, each lasting forty-eight hours. Membership is free and open to all.

AGE ALERT

If a sheath is too restrictive a cut, try a shift. The straight up-and-down style from the 1960s allows you more room to move and groove. But don't completely relive this style by exposing too much skin. Instead, take advantage of the shift's flattering silhouette in a sleeved style with a slightly below-the knee hem.

63

A fitted bodice with stunning details like banding or ruching, a full skirt minus excessive volume, and beautiful accessories like chandelier earrings or a sparkly necklace and a bracelet.

other must HAVES

+ **Maxi dresses**, hemmed to floor length (not longer!) and fitted on top for casual fun

+ **Empire-waist formal column dresses**—a fitted look for those with hips

+ **Evening separates**—for maximum manipulation geared toward your body type

IT'S A STEAL

I love new opportunities for designer discounts. The new sister site to www.revolveclothing.com is www.reverse-reverse.com—it offers prices up to 80 percent off. Reverse membership is by invitation only, but it's possible to be invited off the waiting list. Be patient!

RAISING THE BAR

Do you shy away from drop-waist styles because the fabric gets "caught" on your hips? To still achieve the look, wear a roomier cut like a trapeze dress and add a belt that sinks below your natural waistline. For more casual styles, try a thick band; for dressier versions, a fabric or thin belt works best.

SHAPE SAVER

It's such a drag to wear a strapless dress with droopy boobs. Enter the mini miracle workers, Bring It Up Instant Breast Lifts, which provide a nonsurgical way to give your breasts a temporary boost. Place the waterproof adhesive at the top of each breast (up to a size D) and lift to desired height for a perkier placement that will remind you of your youth. Eight adhesives, $19.99; www.bringitup.com.

BEHIND THE SEAMS

Short waist? Big bust? A drop-waist gown is an alternative to a princess ball gown. It makes a torso appear longer and balances out a heavy chest with a long, lean lower half. Look for scoop necklines, vertical piping, and details like pleats or a belt around or below the drop waist. These details enhance the length of the torso and draw the eye up and down the body.

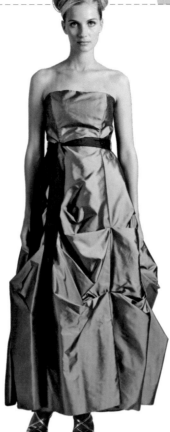

A multitiered skirt that's too short and more prom dress than posh, in a shiny unyielding fabric.

other must LOSE

- **Poofy drop-waist dresses** with draw-string ties

- Thick **coat dresses**

- Dresses with **matching jackets**

- **Full-length evening gowns with tie-dye-appearing ombré,** a gradation of usually monochromatic color from light to dark

sale suckers

Forget the discounted dress that poofs out on the rack. You may love how tiny your waist appears, but an overly full skirt makes you seriously bottom-heavy. Modernize: Go for a shorter skirt (at or above the knee) and say no to strapless. My dream evening designer, Badgley Mischka, has a lower-price line, Badgley Mischka Platinum Label, with perfect dresses to fit the bill.

age alert

The style of this dress is reminiscent of *Gone with the Wind* and is best left at Tara. If you like what a full skirt has to offer—a narrow waist, a supported bust, and covered hips and thighs—find one that's more sleek and tailored, particularly in the torso, in a monochromatic color minus the shine and layers.

temperature falling

How *do* you stay warm in evening attire? I wish I loved dresses with matching jackets or drapey wraps, but I don't. Show creativity; mix and match with pieces you already own. If you're wearing a short full-skirt dress with exposed tulle, try a sleek black leather coat for a rocker vibe. Or go classic with a metallic **save-me** shrug that will match nearly anything. Top Shop has a Premium Beaded Rose Shrug in antique gold, $90; www.us.topshop.com. Beware: No metallic with metallic…too much sparkle.

Sara Blakely, the founder of Spanx, knows a thing or two about smoothing silhouettes. A decade ago, when she couldn't find footless pantyhose, she invented her own. Now she's extended her problem-solving ingenuity to everything from bras to clothing, winning over celebrity fans like Oprah Winfrey and Jessica Alba. With more than 150 figure-saving products to date, Sara shares her shapewear must-haves and tells how to look sensational in your swimsuit.

Generally speaking, what key shapewear pieces should every woman have in her arsenal?

If you like to wear the latest fashions, you are going to need a shapewear wardrobe to match. The most basic shapewear closet should include a mid-thigh shaper to eliminate VPL (visible panty lines) and firm up your lower half under skirts and dresses; footless pantyhose or a capri-length shaper to wear under pants; a high-waisted shaper to cinch the waist and slim the midriff underneath form-fitting dresses, a smoothing cami to eliminate bra lines and bulges in clingy tops; and a full-coverage, high-compression bodysuit for those moments when you need to shimmy into the perfect dress.

If you are on a budget, what is the *one* piece you should have in your closet?

Shaping camis and tanks are great for taming the tummy and providing extra coverage in low-rise jeans and pants. There are now many fashionable

choices that have chic details like lace or silk trim, so you can show them off under a blazer or cardigan and no one will know you're wearing shapewear. High-waisted shapers are also a great way to slenderize your midsection, and they work especially well under slim-fitting skirts and dresses.

Is there such a thing as shapewear overkill? Can you wear too many pieces at once?

As long as you're comfortable, I don't think so. A lot of women wear multiple smoothing pieces at once, like our Bra-llelujah bra under a cami with a girl-short shaper on bottom. A lot of celebrities have admitted to wearing two pairs of Spanx Power Panties at once—I call that commitment. We also have a new line called Skinny Britches, which is a collection of super thin shapers that can be layered for added compression and control. Now celebrities aren't the only ones double Spanx-ing!

If you find yourself between two sizes—say the medium is sausage-squeezing tight and the large is fitted but a little loose—which should you buy?

If neither size fits, that product isn't right for you. I would suggest trying something else.

With most shapewear packaged and not returnable once opened, how can you be sure you're buying the right fit?

Use the size charts and stay true to your size. Sometimes women seeking extra control or added comfort purposely choose the wrong size and end up sacrificing function and comfort. Pinching and rolling are signs of poor fit. If your shaper is rolling up from the leg or down from the waist, you've likely gone with the wrong size. For hosiery shapers, if you are right on the line in between sizes, size down for more compression and up for more comfort. When possible, try before you buy and make sure you can move comfortably in it. I always give our new products the disco test—if I can dance in it and it stays in place, then it's disco approved and good to go!

You recently launched a line of slimming swimsuits. What's your best swimsuit style advice for the most common body types?

If you are tall with a narrow torso, tankinis are your most flattering option because the flare at the hip adds curves to a long frame. Pear shaped? Draw attention to your top, not your hips, with a one-piece bandeau with ruffles. Halter-style one-pieces offer maximum support and are your best bet if you're busty. Petites with a small chest should try a two-piece to elongate their torso, with embellishment on top to give the illusion of a bigger bust. Tummy trouble is best concealed with one-piece styles that have ruching through the midriff— which makes waists look cinched—and/or color blocking with a dark color across the stomach to narrow the waistline and flatten the tummy. Flatter broad shoulders with a deep V-neck one-piece that draws the eye up toward the neck and slims shoulders.

Does the Spanx bikini magically hold you in?

The bikinis in the collection aren't designed to give a ton of slimming compression. They have smart features like leg openings that don't dig in and some light tummy control in the bottoms, but no, they aren't going to magically slim your middle like the one-pieces do. They're just really cute and figure-flattering.

Spanx also offers a swim dress—a swimsuit with an attached skirt. What body type best rocks this look?

The swim dress is perfect for a woman who loves her upper body but wants a little extra coverage through the tummy and down below at her hips.

You're in the dressing room and have tried on a pile of suits, but none of them fit. Help!

Save yourself a headache and use the Spanx swimsuit sizing chart below which works for most swimsuit brands. Based on the measurements in inches of your bust, waist, hips, and torso, you can quickly and painlessly decode your

swimsuit size, which is typically one size larger than your pant size.

Swimsuits can be pricey, especially Spanx suits. How do you make them last?

Our suits are made from a luxurious Italian jersey fabric so that they stay in great shape season after season. Be sure to hand wash them and never put them in the dryer.

You are constantly revolutionizing the industry with innovations, from sexy body suits to Spanx for Men. What new technologies can we look forward to that are making shapewear better than ever?

Invisible shapewear! We are launching a collection of nine classic tops that have invisible shaping built inside, called On Top and In Control. I was inspired to make classic tops that women can wear every day with everything from pencil skirts and heels to jeans and flats. As a new mom on the go, I'm all for anything that easily and comfortably gives me extra control and added style!

SWIM-SUIT SIZE	4	6	8	10	12	14	16
	XS	S	M	M	L	L	XL
BUST	31–32½″	33–34½″	35–36½″	37–38½″	39–40½″	41–42½″	43–44½″
WAIST	23½–25″	25½–27″	27½–29″	29½–31″	31½–33″	33½–35″	35½–37″
HIPS	35–36″	37–38″	39–40″	41–42″	43–44″	45–46″	47–48″
TORSO	58–59″	59½–60½″	61–62″	62½–63½″	64–65″	65½–66½″	67–68″

wear

A skirt suit with a tailored jacket that fits seamlessly over hips and sleeves that end just past the wrist bone, in a flattering dark color like navy, charcoal gray, or black.

+ A single-breasted or single-button style, which is universally flattering

+ Unstiff fabrics like cotton-poly blends and stretch (if you're curvy, structured fabrics like linen and cotton twill)

+ Details that add personality: grosgrain trim, trumpet skirts, flattering pleats, conservative slits

+ A collar to match face shape: bigger face, bigger collar; smaller face, smaller collar

+ A suit skirt showing leg, creating the illusion of length if petite, resting at or slightly above the knee

+ A fitted jacket ending below the waist if you're curvy showcases the waist while grazing over stomach and hips

+ A longer suit jacket to balance leg length if you're tall

MATCH POINT

Maximize suit style with a unique blouse in a gorgeous print or a tie-neck top. It offers a tailored look, especially when the tie ends float down the bodice, creating length. This is the perfect alternative to an overly ruffled blouse, but is not an option for someone with a short neck—it cuts you off.

SHAPE SAVER

Suits that have stretch are God's gift to the working woman. They are comfortable but also form fitting. Look for labels that list elastomers like spandex or Lycra, or literally say "stretch." I love a fabric with a little give to make a professional work suit have that much more *inner* appeal.

IT'S A STEAL

Select your sizes and favorite brands from 625 designers (like Tory Burch, Theory, Fendi, and Anne Klein) at www.Shopittome.com and receive free Salemails via e-mail on suits and other items that go on sale in your size.

SOLE MATES

The obvious choice is a T-strap, loafer heel, or power pumps to complete your professional look, but textured hose or tights are an unexpected twist that adds spice and character. Hue and Wolford hosiery are all available at www.barenecessities.com.

- Double-breasted styles (unless you are flat-chested)
- Fabrics with sheen like satin, which make you look unnecessarily wider
- Unproportional separates (such as a coat that is far wider than its bottom)
- Stiff fabrics that are unyielding (unless you are well proportioned)
- Item described as a "suit" that is more casual wear (as in velour suits or jumpsuits)
- Nehru collars, which close off the neck and make you look like a turtle

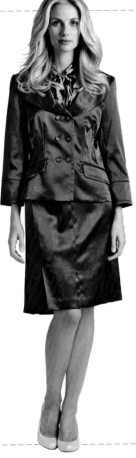

A shiny suit of synthetic material with a boxy double-breasted jacket that's too short in the arms, and a tie-neck blouse that competes with the collar.

outsourcing

If you've been dry cleaning your suit pieces separately to save money, you shouldn't; there will be discoloration between the two pieces and it will be time to toss. Always clean a suit in its entirety so the separates "age" together.

it's a steal

Find it hard to compare various suit styles? Shopstyle.com is a search engine for all things fashion, including suits. Pick your category and view hundreds of mini photos to compare, with designer, price, and store info visible in pop-up boxes. Click on a favorite suit and the site takes you straight to the online retailer to purchase.

shape saver

When it works, double-breasted suiting can help boost the chest of the less-endowed and offer petite frames a bit more stature. A double-breasted military jacket with a V-neck shows just a hint of skin and opens up this style. Look for cute options from Lauren by Ralph Lauren and Thakoon.

shining moment

Do not wear ultra-long dangling earrings or oversized hoops; they compete with the neckline. Keep earrings modest—play it safe with studs (for small face shapes) or small to mid-size hanging earrings (for medium or larger face shapes). Clanging bangles or metallic bracelets are unprofessional. Generally, a necklace that falls past the opening of the jacket collar is just too long.

wear

A neutral-hue suit with a deep V-cut in the fitted jacket, a top button under the bust, and a fabric that fits without creasing in the crotch.

other must HAVES

+ **Pinstripe pantsuits**
+ **Suits with black and white color blocking** that flatter the figure
+ **Color suits** that complement your skin tone

RAISE THE BAR

The deeper the V in your jacket's cut, the more room you have to play with a colorful blouse, a detailed bow, or a ruffled camisole. (See p. 73 for **save-me** shirt choices.) The jacket fabric should be thin enough that you can move and groove without worrying about bunching underneath.

BEST BETS

Designers like Theory, Jones New York, Elie Tahari, Nine West, and Calvin Klein have extensive collections of suits to inspire.

SHINING MOMENT

For contemporary jewelry that is workplace appropriate and still awes, try Katy Beh (www.katybeh.com).

80 percentage of women who wear the wrong bra size

A poorly ~~fitting~~ double-breasted pantsuit in a thick, stiff ~~fabric~~, paired with full-cut pants and a ruffled blouse that chokes the neck.

other must LOSE

- **Heavy brocades, boiled wool or bouclé** that bulk you up like a hockey player
- **Corduroy suits**
- **Velvet jacquard suits**
- **Suits with thick pants** that add weight to thighs and legs

ditch it

For those who are fuller on top, the double-breasted style will make you look even bigger. The result is a shapeless silhouette that screams stuffy rather than chic.

behind the seams

Houndstooth, like herringbone and other tweeds, is a textile pattern often mentioned in classic suiting. Originating in Scotland, this pattern consists of two-tone checks that are either broken or jagged. Traditionally made of wool cloth (but also occasionally cotton and silk), it can be thick, depending on the density of threads, and therefore challenging to wear. Try to find a weave that is thin and thus more conforming to your body shape.

sale suckers

Ten years ago, my mother bought me DKNY suit separates because of the price. The pants were size 10, the jacket, size 4. We took in the pants but they never fit right. I *just* donated the unworn suit to Dress for Success (www.dressforsuccess.org). Another likeminded charitable organization, Bottomless Closet (www.bottomlesscloset.org), repurposes suits and work attire for job-seeking women in need. Lesson learned: Never allow someone to do your suit shopping for you.

wear

An ultra-feminine skirt suit in a bold color that has clean lines and pretty details, like poof sleeves, flounced ruffles, unique belting, or textured fabric.

other must HAVES

+ **Lightweight tweed skirt suits** paired with soft silk blouses

+ **Pretty separates** that work together as an ensemble

+ **Beaded or jewel-toned skirt suits** for evening

MATCH POINT

Are you a girly girl? Play with feminine tailoring…a sweet belt, soft ruffles, delicate sleeves, pretty piping, fabric-covered buttons, and color. Look for skirts with sewn-in lace underlays that peep out from the skirt's hem, and scalloped or asymmetrical hemlines. Avoid overly detailed pockets that will load pounds onto hips.

IT'S A STEAL

Yearn for independent designer duds like Mint by Jodi Arnold, Alice & Olivia, and Trina Turk, at a quarter of the retail price? Thread Lounge Designer Sample Sales (www.threadlounge .com) offer pop-up shops throughout the United States (Dallas, Palm Beach, Houston, and others) for two weeks at a time, year-round. There are also three permanent store locations: two in San Francisco and one in Chicago.

BEST BETS

If we're talking classic, feminine suiting, you can't go wrong with Rebecca Taylor, Armani, or Albert Nipon. For slightly sexier cuts, Bebe offers a wide variety of suits organized by fabric at www.Bebe.com > Shop By Collection > Suiting.

RAISING THE BAR

Check out crisp Farinaz shirting for under suits at www.farinaz.com.

other must HAVES

+ **Tuxedo suits**

+ Tailored, seamed **peplums**
(a straight-cut bodice with a
seam at the waist attached to
a ruffle)—very structured, *tres*
sleek)

A boyish suit with
masculine detailing:
straight cut pants
and a crisp,
tailored jacket.

WELL SUITED

The **save-me** shirt choices to
go under your suit jacket:

V-NECK WITH COLLAR

wear Blouses that are
delicately ruffled, crew neck,
scoopneck, pin-tucked, or
collared shirts

toss Shirt collar that exceeds
the width or proportion of the
jacket collar; V-neck shirt that
plunges lower than the jacket's
V-neck

SCOOP NECK

wear Blouse with detail at
the neck (such as lace or a
ruffle) to showcase the scoop
neck of the jacket

toss Collared shirt

NEHRU COLLAR, BUTTONED

wear No blouse necessary;
an inner shell is a better choice

toss Turtleneck, mock turtle, or
funnel neck—anything that competes with the high-cut Nehru

DOUBLE-BREASTED

wear Crisp collared shirt—
keep it simple

toss Anything too busy, like a
ruffled blouse

RAISING THE BAR

The influence of menswear
in women's fashion is most
evident in women's suiting options, particularly in fall collections. This style reveals its European influence with slimmer and
trimmer cut jackets and pants,
and is an ideal fit for a slender
petite or a narrow frame.

MATCH POINT

This style sports a sophisticated, androgynous look for
power players at work, and
is best accompanied by a
buttoned-up shirt. Keep the
shirt collar within the jacket
for a truly sharp statement.

SOLE MATES

Given the skinny na-
ture of this pant, stick
with pointy-toe styles.

73

wear

A three-quarter-length coat in a classic, fitted shape and neutral color with flattering pockets and cuffs that land at the wrists.

+ A lapel that's face framing—it should be the opposite of your face shape. If you have a heart-shaped or square face, consider a rounded lapel to soften your facial structure. If your face is round or oval, a defined lapel will complement with its angles

+ A coat that allows for movement. Nothing should be tight, including the back, front, and rear

+ A length that flatters your legs. If you have thick calves, go for a mid-calf length or longer, bisecting your trouble area

+ Sleeves that bisect your wrists

+ Securely sewn buttons

+ Pockets that don't interrupt clean lines

IT'S A STEAL
Once a year, Loehmann's has an annual coat sale that never fails to deliver, offering coats first at 20 percent off, then upwards of 80 percent off (www.loehmanns.com).

BEHIND THE SEAMS
When shopping, wear a favorite thick sweater to make sure the coat fits. While most designers adjust sizing to reflect what *may* lie beneath, how you layer is a personal preference. Stretch your arms overhead and sit while wearing the coat.

RAISING THE BAR
Basic coats don't have to bore. Have fun with details—a diagonal zipper or one with large teeth, a fringed hem, an asymmetrical lapel, a faux fur–trimmed collar, unusual hardware like clasps, clip closures, and buckles, embroidered pockets, etc.

INSOURCING
For a coat with a straight up-and-down cut, accessorize. Buy a wide belt and cinch at your waist. This gives your silhouette a boost with instant curves and an interesting, eye-catching detail.

- A coat with armholes cut straight down
- A coat that doesn't button, gapes between buttons, or is missing irreplaceable buttons
- A double-breasted coat if you're busty, petite, or big-shouldered
- A style that requires effort to get in and out of
- Too-short or too-long sleeves
- An uneven hem, that reveals the clothing beneath
- An inner lining that dips below the coat's hem
- A coat that fits you in the shoulders and nowhere else
- A color that washes you out, like yuck green, faded yellow, or pale pink
- A vintage coat that perpetually smells musty

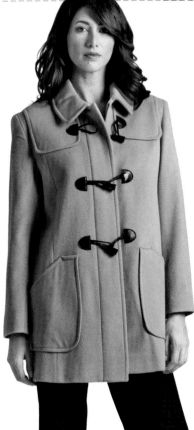

An oversized coat with seams that exceed shoulders, paneling or pockets that crowd the design.

sale suckers

A bargain coat in a funky color might catch your attention at the store, but make sure you really love it outside of the dressing room. Keep in mind that a coat needs to pair with most of your wardrobe—not just your enthusiastic attitude.

temperature falling

Down jackets, coats, and parkas are staples of cold climate urban living, but *can* make you look like a walking sleeping bag. Avoid horizontal quilting that makes you appear wider. Instead, look for a tailored waist and/or a belt to give you some semblance of a silhouette. For warmth, go for a waterproof shell—wet down stinks. Trust The North Face, a high-performance outerwear company that uses the latest fabric technology and *also* has a sense of style: www.thenorth-face.com > women's > jackets & vests > W Triple C Jacket in white or W Atlantic Jacket.

behind the seams

Down is made of the very fine feathers that insulate birds, and is a superb insulator in jackets. Read coat labels to find the "fill power" number, which can range from 500 to 900. Generally, the higher the fill power, the warmer and better the down quality.

wear

A double-breasted and belted trench with signature styling like a notched collar, wrist straps, and side pockets, punched up in plaid for a fresh take.

other must HAVES

+ **Belted camel coats**
+ **Robe tie coats**, which mimic a robe's relaxed comfort in a cozy, fitted sweater knit

SHAPE SAVER

If you are curvy, a belted coat is the easy answer, bringing you in at the waist to play up your greatest assets. Avoid details that draw eyes to your curves—embellished or big pockets or a low-slung belt, for example.

RAISING THE BAR

Trenches are rooted in history and thus adored, stylishly protecting you from the elements. While mid-calf was the length during World War I (and is still considered a traditional length), hemlines have since hiked higher, offering a nice option for those with great gams. Trenches of every color, fabric—from cotton to wool gabardine, from leather to denim (thanks, Tracy Reese!)—and cut (Mint by Jodi Arnold makes a short sleeve) are available.

IT'S A STEAL

Designer Charlotte Russe makes a darling, super short trench coat with classic detailing on the shoulder straps, wrist cuffs, and belt for a bargain $34.99; charlotterusse.com. I adore designer Erin Fetherston, and her line, Edition by Erin Fetherston for QVC.com, is chicly adorable and price-tag accessible, including a classic trench with box pleat detailing for $111. Spanish import Zara always offers sophisticated seasonal coats and jackets, like a feminine trench with notched collar and puff sleeves for just under $80; www.zara.com.

BEHIND THE SEAMS

Thomas Burberry, founder of Burberry and inventor of gabardine (a tough, tightly woven fabric), designed the original trench coat during World War I as a lighter alternative to military coats of the day.

A shapeless crinkle leatherette trench with an enormous collar, in a wide, unflattering cut, in a color that's best reserved for emergency vehicles.

other must LOSE

- **Trenches with oversize belts** or ties that bulk the waist

- **Trenches with serious shoulder pads, flaps, and straps**–makes you a modern-day Inspector Gadget

- **Iridescent polyester trenches**

sale suckers

Usually, trench coat fabrics like cotton drill or poplin are stiffer, so they offer structure to softer frames and make any silhouette ultra-polished and sophisticated. When designers create polyester or leatherette trenches, they disappoint because the crispness and angle disappear and are replaced with a sloppy, formless shape.

ditch it

The best attributes of a terrific trench can also work against you. Overly large pleated flap pockets can bring weight to your midsection and studs along shoulder straps look like spiky shoulder pads.

raising the bar

I don't advise wearing a trench that presents a softer silhouette. If you insist on doing so, then make sure your lower half contrasts with crisp tailoring: menswear pants, fitted trousers, sharp-looking boots. The same principle is true for more masculine-cut outerwear: don feminine separates below.

wear

The tailored boyfriend blazer with rolled sleeves and small shoulder pads for definition, that just covers the bottom, for a long, lean look.

other must HAVES

+ Fitted, women's-cut **blazers**
+ **Boyfriend coats** (even longer than a blazer) that land mid-thigh at longest
+ **Vintage blazers**
+ **Sweater coats**
+ **Swing-back coats**

BEHIND THE SEAMS

The boyfriend blazer is aptly named because it looks as if you stole it from your beau's closet. It's casual. It's masculine. It's a girl posing in guy's clothes for super chic street style. The cut on this coat? Generous and roomy. With boyfriend blazers now made for women, you can score a more tailored look (fitted in the shoulders and nipped in the waist), if you choose.

MATCH POINT

If you practice what I preach about pants in Chapter 2, the rule of proportion suggests wearing this slouchy blazer with a more tailored bottom (such as leggings or skinny pants). But you can just as well pull off a complete masculine look with wide-legged, cuffed pants. If you choose the latter, belt the pants for some waist definition or buckle the exterior of the coat to cinch in your silhouette.

SOLE MATES

The blazer is overtly masculine, and a shoe that counterbalances needs to be feminine yet powerful. Think heels, not flats. Try sexy stacked pumps, funky ankle boots, or cut-out sandals with substantial heels.

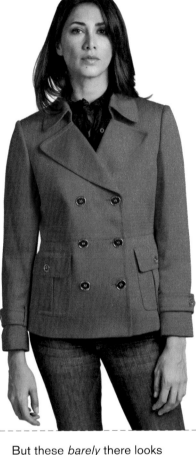

A preppy blazer that hangs too loosely in a double-breasted style that causes the shape of your chest, waist, and shoulders to totally disappear.

other must LOSE

- **Velvet boyfriend blazers**—too much sheen on so much material

- **Checked blazers** in light colors—unflattering

- **All-metallic blazers**—for the chosen few who have the personality of a strobe light

sale suckers

The double-breasted boyfriend blazer is a double negative: ultra boxy and extremely oversized in cut, particularly around the neckline. It's prodigiously square in shape for someone with pronounced shoulders or small bones.

age alert

The ultimate sex appeal of the boyfriend blazer is its bum-skimming qualities—as in *barely* covering the butt over skinny pants or *barely* matching the hem of a short babydoll dress.

But these *barely* there looks are not flirt-appropriate for everyone. For mature audiences, skip the bare legs and pair with fitted pants or a shift dress.

ditch it

If you are petite, this look has got to go unless the blazer is cropped (revealing your waist) and/or somewhat fitted in length so you're not entirely lost. Try La Rok for above-the-waist styles and Kenneth Cole, Vince, and Express for slim and trim cuts.

best bets

Starting at the beginning of October, the first outerwear sales are in full swing, and they extend through January–February. Start with 20 to 25 percent off outerwear from brands like Gap, Urban Outfitters, BCBGMaxAzria, and others.

Slim leather jacket with catchy details like exterior zippers, and a hem that tapers and ends at a flattering point.

other must HAVES

+ Elegant **long leather coats**
+ Leather **biker jackets**
+ **Leather cycle jackets** with asymmetrical zippers
+ Leather **vests**
+ Belted burgundy **leather trenches**

BEHIND THE SEAMS

We tend to think of the leather or faux leather jacket in classic colors such as black. Try a different neutral, like gray, cream, taupe, or tan, or something more vivid like blue, red, or green to liven things up.

IT'S A STEAL

Ideeli is a beloved online designer sale site that is free to join and allows you to take advantage of 80 percent off designer fashion, beauty, and home items. Sales last a mere thirty-six hours or until sold out, with additional seven-hour pop-up sales for the truly spontaneous shopper (www.ideeli.com).

INSOURCING

Caring for leather is essential. In return, it can last a near fashion eternity. Snow Proof is a product by Fiebing that has been around for more than a century. Try the odorless, colorless Snow Proof Weatherproofing Conditioner for waterproofing and restoring smooth leathers, $3.29; www.fiebing .com or www.amazon.com.

BEST BETS

A splurge: Self-described as the most comfortable luxury travel collection for men and women, Ever (www.ever-us .com > online shop > women > jackets) is your rocking source for a black leather jacket that, when paired with a white shirt and jeans, will make you look like you mean business. Fans include Sienna Miller, John Mayer, and Rihanna.

A bomber jacket with bulky features like flap pockets, a bubble torso cut, and thick ribbing on the waist and cuffs.

other must LOSE

- Super **fringed leather jackets**
- Ultra **faded jean jackets**

sale suckers

Leather jackets come in many different styles…but maybe they shouldn't. Watch out for wide ribbing, fluffy faux fur–trimmed collars, pilgrim collars, prodigious fold-over collars, super cropped styles, bulky shearling trim, and bubble or tulip silhouettes.

best bets

When buying a leather jacket as a wardrobe staple, try slim-fit cuts. The bulkiness of the style here, which balloons over the torso with ribbing in all the wrong places, will make you look far bigger than you are. Try a body-hugging single- or double-button straight up-and-down cut or, for more edge, an asymmetrical front zip. Avoid poof sleeves, shoulder pads, pleating, and thick, unpliable leathers.

it's a steal

When it's tough to make a decision about *the* right leather coat, rent! Shopitupchic.com, the boutique retailer that doubles as a renter, offers three levels of month-to-month memberships, allowing the rental of three to four articles of clothing at a time. It's perfect for those who like to constantly wear something new or do a trial run of stylish coats before purchasing.

raising the bar

If leather isn't your thing, Vaute Couture (www.vautecouture.com) offers vegan coats—a **save-me** for animal lovers—with net profits benefiting Farm Sanctuary. Also try the UK-cool Vegetarian Shoes, which makes faux leather jackets in a variety of styles (www.vegetarian-shoes.co.uk).

wear

A cute, preppy anorak in a versatile color, with a cinched straight up-and-down cut and flat front pockets.

other must HAVES

+ **Pea coats**
+ Slim and trim **toggle coats**
+ **Faux fur-trimmed parkas**

IT'S A STEAL

Since 1923, London Fog has been a go-to outerwear designer, and made the first raincoat I ever owned. It's a company that has grown with the trends over time and knows how to make a sporty anorak versatile and water-resistant (www.londonfog.com).

RAISING THE BAR

A draw-cord or adjustable waist means you can cinch this sucker to your body. A convertible collar allows you to wear it flap-happy open or seal-the-deal shut—a nice option, depending on the thickness of your neck. Flat pockets mean no additional bulk.

MATCH POINT

An above-the-knee anorak gives you numerous options for your lower half, from pants to jeans, and even a sporty short skirt. Old rules dictated that a coat cover your skirt. These days, your skirt can peep out an inch or so. Don't wear an anorak with a long skirt; your proportions will be thrown off.

toss

A shapeless anorak with a big, distracting collar and elastic or velcro cuffs and closures, in a stale color like mint green, frosty blue, or bubble-gum pink.

hanging rack : coats

other must LOSE

- Pleated **A-line coats**
- Short, tufted **wool coats**
- Overly puffed-up **puffer coats**

sale suckers

With elastic and velcro, you're bound to feel restricted at some point. Elastic is a cost-cutting manufacturing method that causes itchy cuffs and cuts off circulation. Look for styles that are adjustable with a drawstring for a look that's more smoothly cinched to your body.

ditch it

If you want to slim thighs and hips, this is *not* the look for you. With pockets on the hip and a cavernous cut from the waist down, this coat will make you look twice as wide. Just because an anorak is a cover up on a windy or chilly day, don't think of it merely as something to get you from point A to point B. People can still see you!

age alert

Nothing dates you more than a bubble-gum pink or minty green windbreaker from the '80s. Want to look like you're part of Olivia Newton John's "Let's Get Physical" video? Fine. Have your aerobics and your anorak with matching pants, too—but promise you'll work out to your VHS at home.

shoe rack

How many times have you hurriedly gotten dressed in the morning, wondering which shoe goes with a wide-legged pant? A super-short skirt? Skinny jeans? It's when you're in a time crunch that your shoe knowledge runs out the door—without you—and you wish you had the ultimate guide to dictate your perfect pair.

shoe anatomy

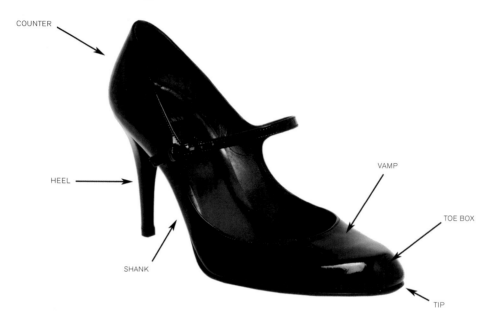

COUNTER

HEEL

SHANK

VAMP

TOE BOX

TIP

SHAPE SAVER

Pointy-toe shoes are ideal for slimming your feet and are guaranteed to lengthen your look. But beware: Seriously pointy "wicked witch" shoes can pose a tripping hazard and decrease circulation in your pinky toes.

SHAPE SAVER

Round and square toes keep leggy legs in check and hide big feet.

break this rule!

Wearing opaque tights with peep-toe shoes is fine.

RAISING THE BAR

Tradition dictates that peep toes are too revealing for a conservative workplace, but that's a rule that's gathered dust. I say, "Wear 'em!" If you're still a little wary, try pairing your peep toe with similar-color opaque or patterned tights.

heels by toe

pointy toe

SLIDE ON WITH: Tailored, slim dress pants or jeans for when you need definition beyond the cuff; simple silhouette dresses; skirts that fall around the knee.

DON'T PAIR WITH: Mini skirts and short shorts because they draw attention to legs—for the wrong reasons.

round toe

SLIDE ON WITH: Nearly everything—this is a very versatile style. Round toes pair with many styles because they have a softer, more feminine look.

DON'T PAIR WITH: Short legs—they'll make your feet look stubby.

square toe

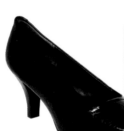

SLIDE ON WITH: Nearly everything, but especially with menswear-inspired ensembles, tweeds, and sharper cuts.

DON'T PAIR WITH: Short legs—like the rounded toe, these will not flatter your feet.

peep toe

SLIDE ON WITH: Nearly anything—a pantsuit or skirt suit during the day, jeans for play, evening dresses for night.

DON'T PAIR WITH: Sheer stockings or toes that you want to hide.

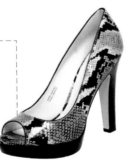

heels by style

stacked

SLIDE ON WITH: A fuller skirt or flared dress pants with wide cuffs—the wider the cuff, the thicker the heel should be. Ideal for balancing curvier frames.

DON'T PAIR WITH: Tailored, slim dress pants or a pencil skirt—this heel will overwhelm their delicacy.

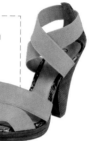

7x

The amount of pressure a three-inch heel puts on the ball of the foot

stiletto

SLIDE ON WITH: A cocktail dress, the ultimate match. Other great options are dress pants and fitted boot-cut jeans for glam appeal.

DON'T PAIR WITH: A mini skirt—the shortness of the skirt and the spike of the heel will leave you overly exposed.

platform

SLIDE ON WITH: Dressy clothing when the heel is polished or casual clothing when the heel is made of cork, wood, or leather.

DON'T PAIR WITH: Delicate, wispy materials or bell-bottom pants.

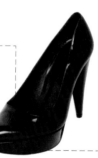

BEHIND THE SEAMS
A stacked shoe heel is made of several layers of material, such as wood or leather, and is usually of medium or heavy thickness.

IT'S A STEAL
The queen of the stacked heel at less-than-royal prices is Jessica Simpson. This singer turned designer flipped her love for shoes into season after season of hot footwear collections that we can actually afford (www.jessicasimpson collection.com).

DITCH IT
Stilettos are the pointiest, slimmest, and (arguably) the sexiest of all heels. But if you have a large frame, this heel is too thin for you—it visually adds pounds above by being so narrow below.

OUTSOURCING
A shoemaker can shorten heels for about $20. Just make sure the overall balance of the shoe doesn't change from front to back.

heels by style

louis

The curviest of all heels, the Louis tapers in the center and flares at the top and bottom, making it very shapely and feminine. It ranges in thickness from skinny to substantial.

SLIDE ON WITH: Items with a similar vibe—it's perfect with a feminine, flirty ensemble.

DON'T PAIR WITH: Heavy tweed fabrics and loose, draped clothing.

kitten

The high heel's comfy cousin, the kitten only hikes up to two inches while still giving you a gentle boost in height. This is generally as tall as a nervous heel-wearer should go especially if merely looking at sky-high stilettos (four inches and higher) makes your ankles shake.

SLIDE ON WITH: Any hemline.

DON'T PAIR WITH: An outfit that needs height to work. A long evening gown is the wrong fit for a kitten heel, as are to-the-floor tailored jeans.

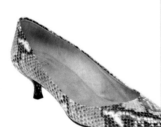

mule

A closed-toe shoe with an open counter or back, mules *classically* feature a high heel. They are the trickiest shoes to walk in because they lack heel support.

SLIDE ON WITH: Trousers or a medium-length skirt, especially if you have hot feet. (Ah, you think I'm kidding!)

DON'T PAIR WITH: A short hemline or thick ankles.

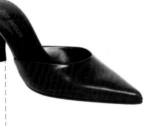

INSOURCING
Keep from ruining the heel of your shoe when driving with Shoe Angels adhesive protectors. Simply apply the reusable stickies to the back of your heel where it hits the car mat to prevent scuffing and damage (not for use on suedes and snakeskins). Place in its chic designer case and store in your glove compartment between uses. $19.95 for 14 Angels and storage case; www.myshoeangels.com.

SHAPE SAVER
For those days when you need a pair of **save-me** shoes after a long day in heels, try Footzy Rolls—rollable ballet flats that are stored inside a tiny bag and fit into your purse, diaper bag, or briefcase… only to reappear when your other shoes are killing you. They come in various colors, $25 each; www.footzyrolls.com.

heels by strap

slingback

SLIDE ON WITH: A monochromatic skirt suit for a sophisticated edge. If the slingback is closed-toe, consider elegant dresses; if the slingback is a sandal, then casual attire works—think wrap shirts and laid-back strapless dresses.

DON'T PAIR WITH: A busily patterned dress, which creates too much visual competition; stockings of any kind; slacks, which hide the heel's gorgeous detail.

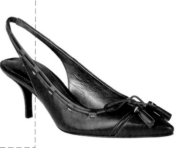

ankle strap

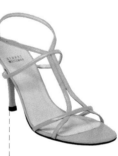

SLIDE ON WITH: A three-quarter-length dress.

DON'T PAIR WITH: Long pants, as the ankle strap gets lost. (Aside from securing your heel in your shoe, what's the point?)

t-strap

SLIDE ON WITH: Any hemline that shows this shoe off (the thicker the straps, the weightier your clothing fabric should be; the more delicate the straps, the lighter it should be).

DON'T PAIR WITH: Pants, which cover the good that a T-strap intends to do.

RAISING THE BAR
The slingback is another strappy style with sex appeal. It reveals the heel and lengthens the legs while remaining a comfortable work choice.

DITCH IT
Ankle straps are not the style of choice for those with short legs. They interrupt the body's vertical line and make you appear even shorter.

SHAPE SAVER
Considered universal **save-me** shoes, the T-strap divides and conquers the foot. For a wide foot, it breaks up the width of skin, while for a narrow foot, the strap adds dimension.

casual heels

oxford

SLIDE ON WITH: Menswear-inspired pieces or ensembles, such as pantsuits, for a snazzy look.

DON'T PAIR WITH: Anything too short or feminine, like a skirt suit. A few can pull off shorts, opaque tights, and oxfords, but most of us should avoid this look.

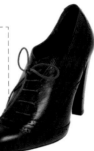

wedge

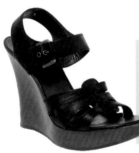

SLIDE ON WITH: Wide-cut pants or shorts with a little flare, summer dresses, fuller skirts—a wedge best balances curvier frames.

DON'T PAIR WITH: Skinny cropped pants, as it makes feet look enormous.

mary jane

SLIDE ON WITH: Relaxed-fit pants, skirts that fall at the knee or are three-quarter-length

DON'T PAIR WITH: Slim-cut pants or socks—unless you're attempting a 1950s flashback.

BEHIND THE SEAMS
Oxfords were named after the short shoes with laces or buckles, historically called half-boots, worn by students at Oxford University.

DITCH IT
Avoid a wedge if you are short *and* plus-size, as it will make you look wider.

BEST BETS
Zappos offers widths ranging from 3E to One Size (OS), and everything in between (www.zappos.com).

IT'S A STEAL
The extensive site www.shoebuy.com has branched into the high-end arena with http://designer.shoebuy.com. From Stuart Weitzman to Bally, Salvatore Ferragamo to Delman, this site showcases something for all, with free shipping on purchases *and* returns. Sort by the "Percent Off" function to see the best deals first: A recent search found golden Miu Miu lace-up flats for 82 percent off the retail price.

RAISING THE BAR
When they're school-girl cute flat, Mary Janes are best suited for casual dressing. Sky-high heeled versions are sophisticated day-to-night options.

dressy flats

patent leather

SLIDE ON WITH: At or above the knee skirts; dressy or evening looks, which complement the luxurious shine of the leather; nearly all jeans aside from extreme flares

DON'T PAIR WITH: Other leather pieces.

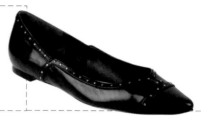

embellished

SLIDE ON WITH: Any unembellished outfit with any hemline, to add zest to your look.

DON'T PAIR WITH: Heavily embellished clothing—matchy-matchy is a no-no.

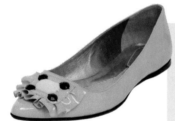

pointy toe

SLIDE ON WITH: A short skirt to lengthen both feet and legs, or perfectly hemmed pants that reveal the shoe's toe.

DON'T PAIR WITH: Opaque tights. Better to go bare than look matronly.

MATCH POINT
Flats *generally* don't jive with three-quarter length skirts that fall below the knee. Because of the lack of heel height, they make your legs look short and you look stumpy.

SOLE MATES
In warmer weather, flats and fitted capri or cropped pants are the best of friends.

RAISING THE BAR
Wide feet a problem for you? Wear pointy-toe flats to make your feet appear narrower. And although ballet flats—modeled after a ballet slipper with a thin sole, short to no heel, and traditionally, drawstring ties—are versatile for dressy or casual occasions, avoid them in your case, as they will make your feet appear to "spill" out.

SHAPE SAVER
Since 1958, Hush Puppies (www.hushpuppies.com) has produced comfortable footwear, and now does so with stylish flair. Search for shoes using the size and width feature (from narrow to extra wide) and check out chic metallic flats in their Soft Style line.

92

casual flats

loafer

SLIDE ON WITH: Classic cut straight-leg or slightly flared trousers for a trendy menswear-influenced look.

DON'T PAIR WITH: Bare feet—wearing loafers without socks was trendy in the '80s, but it's all about socks now (try them rolled low for a geek-chic look).

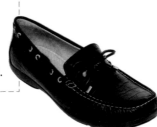

flip flop

SLIDE ON WITH: Jeans, cutoffs, shorts, or casual summer dresses—and don't forget polished toes and moisturized heels.

DON'T PAIR WITH: Dressy outfits—and never on your wedding day! Get a cute, flat bridal shoe for dancing.

fashion sneaker

SLIDE ON WITH: A casual outfit—they are über sporty.

DON'T PAIR WITH: Work or evening attire. Keep in mind, anything that looks remotely like a gym sneaker needs to be relegated to the gym only!

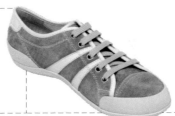

INSOURCING
Need some height without the heel? Try Women's LiftKits shoe lift inserts in a closed shoe and increase your height by up to two inches (www.myliftkits.com).

9 out of 10 women wear shoes that are too small for their feet

DITCH IT
Slides, which include close-toe, open-heel sneakers, are a tough sell for me: The chunky, heavy look doesn't improve the look of ankles, calves, or feet, and is a particular eyesore if you have dry, cracked heels. (See Chapter 8 for the ultimate heel-repairing, at-home pedicure scrub.)

boots

under the knee

SLIDE ON WITH: Nearly everything. It is the go-to **save-me** option for women, as it slims the calf.

DON'T PAIR WITH: Knobby or chunky knees. Because of where this boot ends, it draws attention to that area.

mid-calf

SLIDE ON WITH: A shorter hemline to create leg length.

DON'T PAIR WITH: A knee-length skirt, as this boot bisects your calves at the meatiest part of the muscle, making uncovered legs look stumpy.

ankle/peep toe

SLIDE ON WITH: Skinny leggings or opaque tights in a matching (for playing safe) or bright (for making a statement) color, jeans tucked into the boots, frilled dresses that end at the knee and miniskirts.

DON'T PAIR WITH: Cropped or capri pants, cocktail dresses, skirts or dresses that hit below the knee if you have shapely calves.

over the knee

SLIDE ON WITH: Dark, opaque tights, tucked-in leggings or jeans, skirts or dresses that fall a few inches from the top of the boot.

DON'T PAIR WITH: Skirts or dresses that hit right at the top of the boot. And beware if you dare to go bare—thighs might look larger than you'd like.

BEST BETS
Nine West (www.ninewest .com) changes up designs each season. A current web site tab smartly sorts "Boots Under $99" for those on a budget. Elizabeth and James has fashionable options from over the knee to wedge booties.

DITCH IT
Muscular calves? The mid-calf is not the boot for you. Opt instead for a knee-high boot for full lower leg coverage.

SHAPE SAVER
Silhouettes, a plus-size clothing company, offers a large range of shoes in wide-calf and wide-width styles, particularly in stylishly to-die-for boots (www.silhouettes.com).

94

boots

rocker/biker

SLIDE ON WITH: The shortest hemline you can muster, with leggings to show off the boots. Skinny jeans also hit the mark for a complete rocker chic ensemble.

DON'T PAIR WITH: Wide-leg trousers, which give too much of a clunky feel on the bottom half.

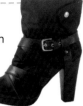

equestrian/riding

SLIDE ON WITH: Leggings and other tailored pants that are tucked into the boot. Also wear with short skirts paired with leggings.

DON'T PAIR WITH: Wide-leg pants or three-quarter-length skirts or dresses, as they look frumpy with flat boots.

western

SLIDE ON WITH: All types of denim, tucked or untucked; long skirts; floral printed frocks; any casual look to rope in the cool factor.

DON'T PAIR WITH: Other Western pieces—the goal is not to look like an actual cowgirl.

RAISING THE BAR
Hunter, designer of the Original Green Wellington rain boot, has been making Wellies since 1856 (www.hunter-boot.com). Today, offshoot styles are reasonably priced, funky, and downright adorable, and are available in nearly every print and pattern, from daisies to Indian-inspired swirls. Try www.Target.com > Shoes> Women's > Rain Boots. Wellies are meant to protect, so don't wear them with short hem lines; instead, tuck, tuck, tuck in those bottoms.

TEMPERATURE FALLING
Don't you hate cold toes? Polar-Wrap's Toasty Feet insoles use advanced aerogel insulation (the stuff NASA astronaut suits are made of) to block both cold and heat, for a moderate temperature for your soles in any season (www.polarwrap.com).

IT'S A STEAL
Restricted Shoes, which caters to teens and women, has rockin' prices on super-sweet styles, including ankle boots, over-the-knee boots, and Western-style boots. Details like laces, grommets (metal-rimmed holes), and buttons up the fun factor. Free UPS ground shipping (www.restrictedshoes.com).

sandals

super strappy

SLIDE ON WITH: Dresses and skirts with tights or bare legs. If heeled, any style of trouser; if flat, cropped pants.

DON'T PAIR WITH: Prints that distract; jeans that you tuck the sandal strap over (this is a recent celeb mishap called "trying too hard"); a mini skirt if your super-strappy sandal is a stiletto.

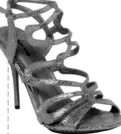

wooden

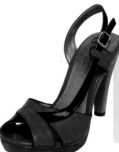

SLIDE ON WITH: Jeans and casual attire, and cropped jeans and higher hemlines if the heel is shorter.

DON'T PAIR WITH: Delicate fabrics, which seriously unbalance the look.

metallic slingback

SLIDE ON WITH: Evening attire with shine or a sexy pair of dark wash jeans.

DON'T PAIR WITH: Knits, which are too heavy for this style. Instead, think delicate fabrics.

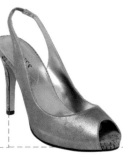

IT'S A STEAL
Seychelles offers every strappy sandal incarnation that you can think of: flat, wedge, heel, thong, and more. The beachy, bright colors, endearing embellishments, and digestible price points are sure to make you smile (www.seychellesfootwear.com).

BEST BETS
For celebrity stylist Rachel Zoe's latest shoe and bag picks, plus free shipping both ways, visit www.piperlime.com.

SHAPE SAVER
Thongs are generally too big if you have low arches, slim, or super narrow feet—you'll be slip-sliding away.

SHAPE SAVER
Laugh if you like, but Smart-Heel's removable heel protector performs a **save-me** on your stilettos every time you walk over a grate or sidewalk seam or cut a curb too close—www.smartheel.com, $11.95 per pair. Who's laughing now?

sandals

shoe rack : sandals

thong

SLIDE ON WITH: A casual long skirt, cropped pants, shorts.

DON'T PAIR WITH: Formalwear.

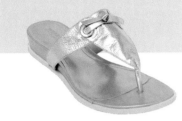

gladiator

SLIDE ON WITH: Casual shorts, jeans, cropped pants, maxi and casual dresses.

DON'T PAIR WITH: Slim-fit three-quarter-length dresses, as these shoes are too spirited for such a serious ensemble.

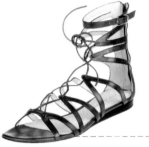

65
Percentage of women age 18 to 49 who haven't had their feet measured for shoes in the past five years

BEST BETS
Te Casan by Natalie Portman is probably one of the most renowned lines of vegan shoes. Her designs, along with other chic vegan/vegetarian options (where no animal leathers or products are used in a shoe's creation) like olsenHaus and Beyond Skin, are available at www.endless.com > women's shoes > vegetarian.

IT'S A STEAL
Payless Shoes (www.payless .com) has signed top designers to create exclusive lines under its label for a fraction of the cost. They include Abaeté, Lela Rose, Christian Siriano, Alice + Olivia, and Zoe & Zac. Fashion-forward, affordable shoes? Sign me up!

IT'S A STEAL
Simply put: great gladiators at Mia (www.miashoes.com).

ethnic

CASUAL

clog

SLIDE ON WITH: Wide-leg pants, an A-line skirt with a hemline at or slightly below the knee.

DON'T PAIR WITH: A hemline that rises above your knees, or anything that gives you a tailored or tapered silhouette, such as a pencil skirt.

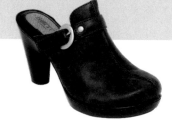

moccasin

SLIDE ON WITH: Jeans.

DON'T PAIR WITH: A fringed suede skirt.

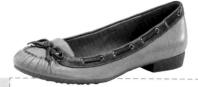

espadrille

SLIDE ON WITH: A three-quarter-length skirt or shorts.

DON'T PAIR WITH: A long skirt, capris, or short legs. Anything that wraps up the calf is a detriment to those who don't have a lot of leg to spare.

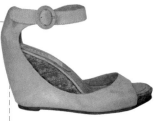

RAISING THE BAR
Think you're a shoe designer? Custom-design your own fancy footwear at www.milkandhoneyshoes.com. While this company specializes in personal appointments and shoe parties in Los Angeles, it also gives you the option to create your shoes online or on the phone. Choose your shoe silhouette, then decide everything from heel height to embellishments and more. Prices vary: flats start at $225, heels $250, platforms $275, vegan $325.

SHAPE SAVER
Skinny feet a problem? Not anymore: Designer Donald J. Pliner specializes in narrow-width shoes (www.donaldjpliner.com).

PAIN-FREE, SAVE-ME FOOTWEAR

shoe rack : comfort

KENNETH COLE 925 TECHNOLOGY SILVER EDITION COLLECTION

Named for its comfort staying power for a 9 to 5 work day, this new extension of the Kenneth Cole brand features an exclusive, patented design, including a double-layered Poron memory foam footbed, flaxseed-filled arch supports, embedded cork, and a sheepskin lining for ultra cush. Look for another signature touch: the silver-toned heels on the pumps, slingbacks, booties, and flats. www.kennethcole.com

TARYN ROSE

Founded by an orthopedic surgeon in 1998, this company of Italian-made, hand-sewn shoes brings a touch of sexy to pumps and high-heel boots. Among the first to use Poron memory foam for cushioning, Taryn Rose doesn't shy away from heels: try three inches-plus on for size! Also look for signature floral embellishments on cute flats. www.tarynrose.com

COLE HAAN AIR

Cole Haan's marriage to Nike Air technology has produced a current Air collection of more than 525 styles of shoes for men and women. Owning these sleek styles, which range from bridal sandals to high-heeled boots, means that with each step, you'll stride in comfort. www.colehaan.com

POUR LA VICTOIRE

The enclosed platforms (not platform sandals), ankle booties, and boots from this brand have generous padding in the ball of the foot, making them shockingly cushy despite their high heights. www.pourlavictoire.com

ANYI LU

Drawing on her experiences as a competitive dancer (and her smarts as a chemical engineer), designer Anyi Lu rumba-ed her way to making beautiful shoes with a ballroom sensibility, meaning they focus on great fit and flexibility. Her shoes feature Poron memory foam, toe boxes that don't scrunch your piggies, and Sachetto construction: the shoe form molds to the foot. www.anyilu .com

DKNYC

Some DKNY styles offer "lightly padded footbeds," which I recommend if you want the ultimate in comfort. www.dkny.com

AEROSOLES

Since 1987, Aerosoles has been synonymous with comfort, incorporating extra cushion, padded footbeds, and flexible rubber soles to a wide range of shoe styles. What's not to love about 3-inch, two-tone peep-toe navy pumps that add spring to your step and knee-high boots with tassels and stud detailing? Both are full of sass and kick, without killing your feet. www.aerosoles.com

87%
of women have suffered due to painful footwear

99

top shelf :
handbags

Why do women love shopping for handbags? Because, unlike clothes, we don't need to shed a thing to try them on. For this reason, the handbag department is one of my favorite quick-stop shopping fixes to instantly add splash to a wardrobe. Still, among those who have "the bag bug," I'm surprised by the number of people who wear them all wrong.

wear

bags of ideal size and shape for tall women

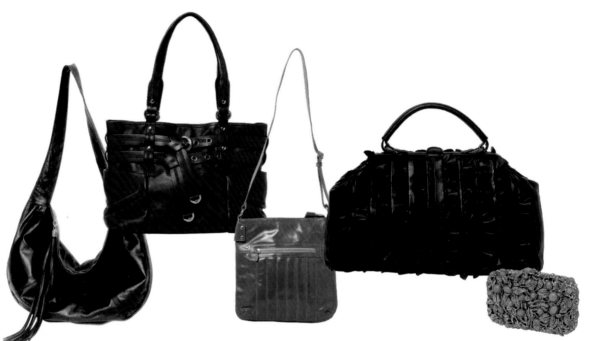

LEFT TO RIGHT: sac, medium to large unstructured shoulder bag, cross-body messenger bag, trapezoid or ruffle satchel with soft curves, hand-held clutch (with body texture such as sequins, gems, rhinestones, etc.)

LENGTH
Your height means you can handle a bag that hits anywhere from the waist to slightly below the hip.

SHAPE
You have the luxury of vertical space to work with, so fill it with medium to larger unstructured bags. You can play with volume.

IT'S A STEAL
An invitation-only online sale site, www.ruelala.com has great accessory sales, including handbags from designers like Marc by Marc Jacobs and Botkier—sometimes 75 percent off and more. Refer a friend who makes a purchase and get a $10 credit toward your account.

RAISING THE BAR
Haven't found a bag you love? Laudi Vidni ("individual" spelled backwards) allows you to custom design your own luxury handbag—and there are 10,000 possibilities. Choose a silhouette, select the interior and exterior fabrics, and decide on hardware options. Prices start at $85. Bags are made in Chicago using soft imported leathers (www.laudividni.com).

bags that don't work for tall women

STYLE TO GO

IF BAGS CONFOUND YOU FOLLOW THESE THREE SIMPLE GUIDELINES.

1. Your bag shape and body shape *shouldn't* match. If you're tall and thin, consider an unstructured, slouchy bag. If you're round and curvy, get a structured style. Think opposite for a beautiful balance. And if you're average all around, lucky you—you can sport any style. Be sure to try your bag on in front of a mirror. It's a must.

2. The bag *should* hit your assets. If you have hips, make sure the bag hits above or below but not *at* your hip. If you are busty, the bag should hit below the bust. If you are petite, your bag should go no lower than the waist or you'll appear to be all bag and no body! Tall? Celebrate your stature with a long bag that hits just below the hip.

3. Consider your bag's main functions. Will you wear it to work? Are you a mom on the go? Do you need a bag to carry you through a weekend or simply to hold a compact, lipstick, and ID for a special evening out? Do you dig pockets or just one main compartment? The answer to these questions will determine the size, style, and durability of your bag. A small crystal clutch won't likely hold a work file…

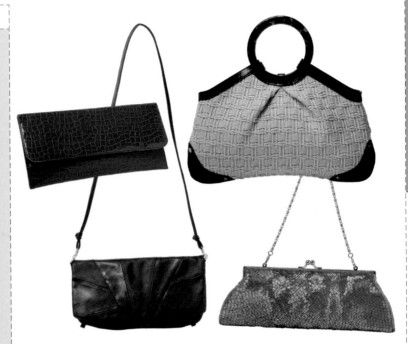

CLOCKWISE FROM TOP LEFT: elongated envelope clutch, top handle bag with strict frame, short-strapped evening bag, über long straps with tiny purse

length

A bag that fits in the crook of your armpit will emphasize your height and make your legs look like beanpoles. If you are tall, you can pull off bags with long straps, as long as the purse isn't tiny—that just makes you appear lanky.

shape

A top handle bag with a strict frame and rigid edges produces a stark overall look and creates too many angles when juxtaposed against a tall frame. Instead, consider a rounded or trapezoid satchel with soft curves to better balance your look.

wear

bags of ideal size and shape for petite women

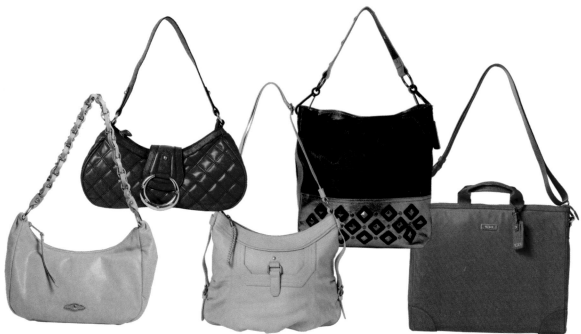

LEFT TO RIGHT: hobo, baguette with strap, bucket bag, small shoulder bag, small to medium handheld briefcase

LENGTH

Because you want to elongate but not overwhelm your frame, the bag should hit anywhere from under your arm to the hollow of your waist. Choose thinner, more delicate straps.

SHAPE

Think proportionally smaller, and don't venture bigger than a medium-size bag. With your body type, bag shape is less of an issue so you can embrace a round or slouchy bag.

SHAPE SAVER

After shelling out money for a handbag, don't you want your purse to keep its shape? Pursendipity is an eco-friendly moldable foam that slips into your bag so it retains the original form: no creases, no folds. It's a little pricey, so reserve it for that special bag you don't want to slouch on the shelf. Available in leopard print or pink: small $44, medium $48, extra large $52; www.pursendipity.net.

BEST BETS

To keep your purse off the floor or off your lap when dining out, use a Luxe Link handbag holder, a chicly designed hook that hangs from a desk or table. Starting at $35; www.luxelink.com.

toss

bags that don't work for petite women

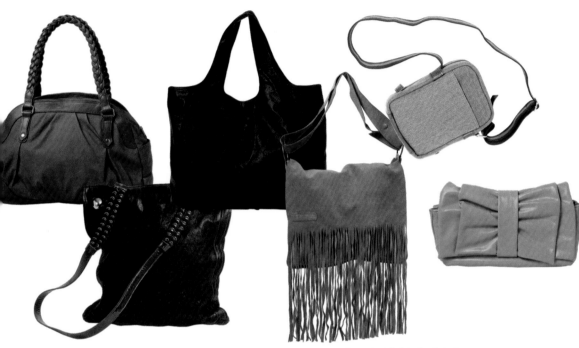

LEFT TO RIGHT: engulfing shoulder bag, cross-body messenger bag (with big body), large tote, drippy fringe bag, pochette, oversized clutch

length

An overly long bag body or strap will make it look like the bag is taking *you* for a walk, as opposed to the other way around.

shape

Enormous bag-size satchels that could literally carry a small child are trendy—but they're not for petites. A too-big bag will envelop you entirely.

$31
the average price of a woman's handbag

105

wear

bags of ideal size and shape for curvy women

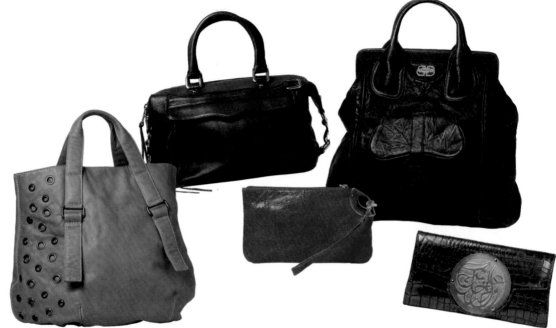

LEFT TO RIGHT: tote, structured, framed satchel, wristlet, square or rectangular shoulder bag, oversized envelope or foldover clutch

LENGTH
Your bag should hit the smallest point of your curves, below the bust and above the hips.

SHAPE
Look for medium to larger bags with structure, form, and stiffer fabrics (firmer leather, canvas, nylon, woven straw) to best complement your frame.

BEST BETS
Buying a pre-owned designer handbag can be nerve-wracking, particularly when you question whether or not it is the real deal. Fashionphile.com is a site to trust. It sells pre-owned luxury handbags primarily on consignment and guarantees each bag's authenticity. The site has a large choice of easy-to-search selections representing the best, from Hermes to Chanel to Louis Vuitton. Don't let the $10,000-plus price tags depress you because there are bags available in the $200 range as well.

ever wonder how much a typical handbag weighs?
Only 3.3 pounds in 2009, down from 7.7 pounds in 2007.

bags that don't work for curvy women

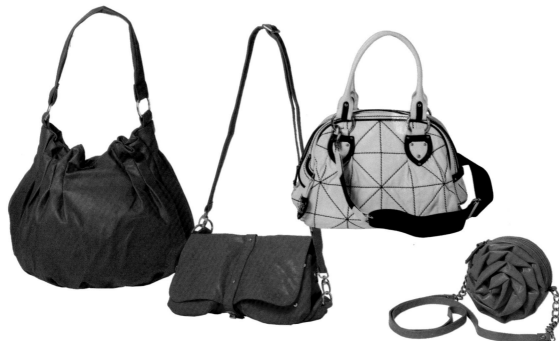

LEFT TO RIGHT: relaxed hobo, full-shape saddle bag, rounded quilted, round or oval minaudieres with strap; rosette evening bag

length

A bag with handles that barely clear the arm will get lost in your armpit. A shoulder bag with long straps is no better because the bag's body will hit at the hip and make you look wider.

shape

Avoid slouchy bags that look like cushioned pillows, round and duffle-shaped bags, structure-less satchels, oval handles, and super thin chain straps.

HANDBAG SITES THAT I LOVE

http://haydenharnett.com
www.mattandnat.com
www.endless.com
couture.zappos.com
www.efashionhouse.com
www.vintage-instyle.com
www.mytheresa.com
www.target.com
www.revivalboutique.com
www.laurenmerkin.com
www.coach.com (Poppy collection)

from the mouths of mavens: LAUREN MERKIN

Lauren Merkin is the Queen of the Clutch. Armed with an MBA from Columbia University and with no previous experience in fashion, she started sewing hand-bags in 2002 and landed her designs at Bergdorf Goodman within a few months. Her coveted handbags—particularly her signature clutches—make a powerfully chic yet timeless statement. It's no wonder that Reese Witherspoon and Selena Gomez flock to her for sophisticated accessories. As CEO of her eponymous brand, Merkin shares her hints for selecting and caring for your bags, and tells why a bookshelf is your best friend for storage in the off-season.

It's a sea of handbags out there. What should women look for when shopping for a new handbag?

The goal is to balance what you love with what you need. Fashion is supposed to be fun, so my first suggestion would be to start with a style or color that jumps out at you and then make sure the functionality works for your life. Does it fit the items you carry daily? Does it feel comfortable to wear? Is it a color that works with most of your wardrobe? Versatility is key.

What beyond-basic bags should we add to our collection?

I would add a more casual clutch to the essentials. Often a true evening bag is quite small, metallic, or embellished. For most nights out, that would be too much. I suggest a larger leather clutch in black or a neutral. I gravitate to gray clutches again and again, especially when I travel, because they are so versatile.

Once you have the essentials, then you can be a little more whimsical in your choices—try unusual colors and funky embellishments, or splurge on that bag you may only use once a year but keep eyeing. Some other beyond-the-basics styles to consider: a medium cross-body bag works well for weekends or travel, a top-handle duffel can add lady-like style, and of course, I think a girl can never have too many clutches!

Speaking of color, what's the best shade to choose when bags come in a rain-bow of choices?

I think some women are afraid of color, but they shouldn't be. The most versatile colors are not al-ways black or brown. We've found that some of our yellow, green, and multicolored bags can match almost any outfit!

Let's talk about materials and what we should look for.

Often it *is* the materials and textures that transform our bag shapes season to season. I have worked with everything from cork and sequins to calf hair and perforated leathers. For clutches I usually gravitate toward lambskins because of their softness, but here, too, there's lots of variety: There are washed, embossed, and embroidered lambskins. Fabrics are a little less durable. For the bags you schlep around daily, I like slightly heavier leathers such as calfskin, buffalo, or cow hides. The skins tend to be a bit thicker and more capable of handling the normal wear and tear.

Do certain bag materials work better for daytime rather than evening?

There are no absolute rules for day vs. night. It really depends on how you put a look together. If you are going to wear sequins for day, then your bag has to be balanced by the rest of your look—that is, don't pair a sequined clutch with a sequined skirt.

What is your best style advice for wearing a purse with a long strap?

I love this trend because it offers so much flexibility. You can wear it on your shoulder or cross-body to be hands-free. If you are going to wear it cross-body, make sure that the strap does not inter-fere or conflict with your outfit. Cross-body straps can sometimes detract from the shirt or necklace you are wearing, so be sure to check yourself out in the mirror before walking out the door.

What is your greatest handbag pet peeve?

Seeing a day bag out on a Sat-urday night! Your day bag should not double as your going-out bag. The most offensive is any oversized, overstuffed bag. You only need the essentials out with you at night. Every woman should invest in at least two classic clutches or evening bags.

You are acclaimed for your clutches. What's your secret for pairing a clutch proportionally to your body type?

Generally speaking, I think clutch-es work for any body type, but the proportion of your clutch should fit your outfit. If you are wearing a casual, more layered look, then a larger clutch works best. A dainty clutch just gets lost. And on the flip side, a more delicate evening look is best paired with a scaled-down clutch.

How can most of us spot the difference between a real designer handbag and a fake?

This can be hard if you don't know what to look for in terms of logos, signature lining and stitching, etc. If you're going to buy a designer bag on eBay, you need to do your research. Make sure the seller has excellent ratings and feedback and that the pictures are clear, not copied from another site. You can't go wrong buying designer bags from high-end web sites like Net-a-porter (a favorite!) and any department store's web site, like Neiman Marcus, Barneys, or Saks.

Do you have stores you like to shop for non-designer bags?

You can find some great non-designer bags in vintage stores. The best ones don't even have labels! What Goes Around Comes Around is an amazing vintage store in New York City, and Etsy.com is a wonderful site for one-of-a-kind finds.

I adore vintage, too. What should I look for in a qual-ity vintage handbag?

Leather tends to dry out over time, so a lot of vintage bags can show cracks. Look for one that has been well cared for and the leather conditioned. Hardware is another element that can deterio-rate over time, so it's important to check that hinges and closures are functioning well.

Most of us don't even think about cleaning our bags. Should we?

Cleaning leather is very tricky and should only be done when abso-lutely necessary. There are a vast number of leathers out there and many have gone through incred-ibly unique tanning processes. Lexol—or any non-darkening conditioner—is one product we recommend. Just be sure to follow the directions for diluting on the back of the package and always test any cleaning product on a hidden spot before treating the rest of the bag. Taking your bag to a professional you trust is often the best way to go.

Any sources for finding a great bag repair shop?

I trust word of mouth and find that most reliable shoemakers do handbag repairs as well.

Any tips and tricks for storing off-season bags?

The ideal way is to stuff the inside with paper to maintain the shape of the bag, and then keep it in a dust bag to protect the exterior. Clutches are a bit easier. I tend to keep them out all year round, organized like books on a bookshelf. A lot of clutches have frames, so I store them upside down with the frame on the shelf for stability.

top shelf : handbags

accessory drawer:
belts

I'll admit (in a hushed whisper) that I've had a bit of a belt phobia my entire life. I always thought I had a belly and felt that belts would unattractively accentuate my middle and my hips. Boy, was I wrong...

wear

A medium-width leather belt, not too tight or loose, smartly placed at the thinnest part of the waist.

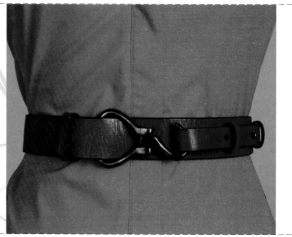

other must HAVES

+ **Snakeskin belts**
+ **Thin patent leather belts**
+ **Vegan belts**

MATCH POINT

Pairing the right belt to your shape and the clothes it services is key. Thin frame? Try a skinny belt (starts at a half-inch) or the most flattering **save-me** for all bodies: the medium-width belt, approximately one to two inches wide, placed a smidgen above your natural waistline. Wear too wide a belt and your proportions will be out of whack.

RAISING THE BAR

A belt shouldn't add bulk. It should define your waist at the narrowest part of your torso, normally bisecting at or slightly above the navel. A hip belt, a.k.a. the hipster, should fall low-slung on the hips like the edge of a low-rise jean (a look best suited for average to short-waisted women).

BEST BETS

It's hard not to find an appealing handmade cincher at B-low the Belt (www.b-lowthebelt .com). Look for attractive grommets, drop ties (two ends of a knotted belt that dangle loosely), studded, and brooch buckle belts…basically, anything but the ordinary.

A poorly sized three-inch or wider patent leather belt that, when secured too tightly, highlights excess pounds at the waist.

other must LOSE

— **Plastic see-through belts** that reveal underlying wrinkles

— **Stretch belts**

— **Lattice belts** with cutouts

— **Cheap elastic belts**

ditch it

Remember that a patent's sheen draws the eye, attracting attention directly to your midriff. Too wide or too shiny a belt on any ensemble can look disproportionate and unintentionally steal the show, particularly if love handles spill over.

insourcing

Though in Chapter 2 I advised you to purge your wardrobe of elastic waistbands, a belt *can* discreetly cover up an unsightly waistband or an unflattering cut on otherwise fabulous pants.

sole mates

Don't pressure yourself into thinking your belt and shoes need to match; for example, a patent belt with patent shoes can be overly synchronized.

ever wonder how belts are sized?

They're measured from the edge of the belt (right before the buckle) to the middle of the holes. Hipster belts are automatically sized to hang lower, so measure just above your hipbone rather than under it.

wear

A thin metallic belt, with or without a buckle adornment, half an inch wide.

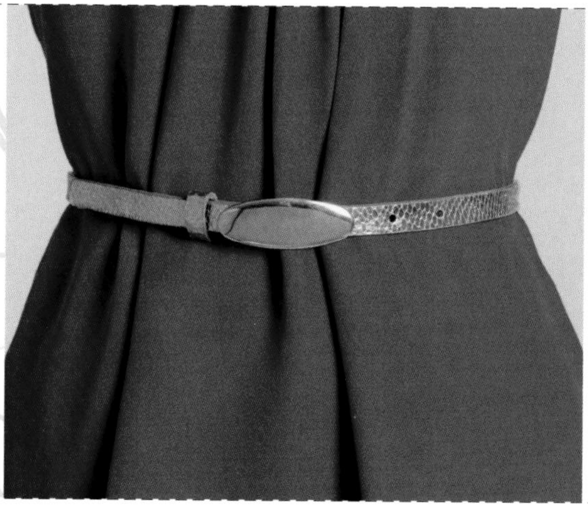

other must HAVE

+ **Monochromatic belts**
+ **Skinny belts** with grommets
+ **Dual pyramid** (it wraps around twice) **skinny belts**

BEST BETS

A great way to embrace a trend is with a belt. Try playing with textures (snakeskin, leathers), prints (animals like leopard), or metallics. Kristin Kahle, Calvin Klein, and Ralph Lauren have tasteful cinchers.

SHAPE SAVER

Because they are thin (sometimes super thin at a quarter of an inch), skinny belts allow you to maximize layering without bulking up, and offer the most options if you like the look of a belt over a jacket, cardigan, and blouse, for example. Skinny belts are particularly good for petite and short-waisted gals as they don't overwhelm.

RAISING THE BAR

Adding a contrasting colored or metallic belt to a monochromatic outfit makes an instant fashion impact, brings attention to your waist, and defines your shape.

MATCH POINT

Metallics shouldn't be paired with like metallics or you'll start to look like you're wearing a spacesuit. Try a metallic belt on a solid-color dress (like black or purple) or a black belt on a metallic dress.

A chain metal belt with numerous hanging pieces that hits and widens the stomach and hips.

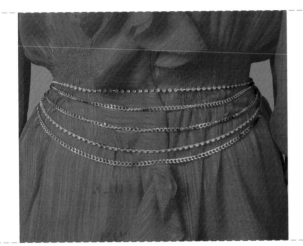

other must LOSE

- **Chain belts** that attach to a wallet
- **Money belts**
- **Fringe belts**
- **Pearls and chains** mixed together

ditch it

Chain belts with multiple strands are not only heavy, they also add baggage. Think about where the chain dangles: If it hits across the stomach, hips, or thighs, you won't be doing yourself any favors.

best bets

The best chain belts have a single body chain and exude tough chic. If you really like the look of dangling strands, limit it to just one. Because this belt is heavy, it looks most natural slung low just below the hipline. Be sure to pair it with a sleek ensemble.

shape saver

It may sound counterintuitive that a single low-slung chain belt offers definition to your silhouette when it hangs loose, but it does. Women with thick midriffs or those who want to lengthen their upper torso just need to buckle lower at the hip. Don't wear this style too tight or the only thing you'll be cinching is yourself—into two unattractive halves.

A double buckle belt with an interesting clasp or detail, worn over a flowy fabric.

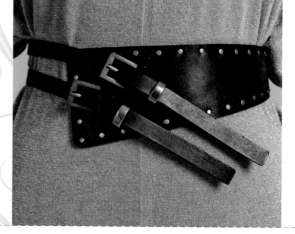

other must HAVES

+ **Single buckle belts** with a double hole for a sleeker look

+ **D-ring belts**

SHAPE SAVER

Tummy trouble? Try a medium to wide belt (wide is defined as two inches or more) to tuck in that tummy and give you a smooth silhouette. A wide belt, in this case, is the ultimate waist-whittling accessory.

IT'S A STEAL

Elegantly Waisted (www.shopbop.com) has belts that run the gamut of designs and widths. Pay particular attention to the selection of unusual textures (like ruffled leather) and tastefully studded and crystal cinchers.

MATCH POINT

Wide cinchers are a fabulous way to define the waist when wearing oversized sweaters, dresses of thinner fabrics, and even shorter jackets. In general, wide belts work with thin or thick fabrics as long as the weight of the material matches the heaviness of the belt. Generally, more volume demands a bigger belt.

RAISING THE BAR

The double buckle belt exudes strappy cool and comes in a variety of styles (woven, braided, canvas, corset). Make sure the buckles align over your stomach; over the hips will unflatteringly widen that area.

A very wide obi-style belt with bulky, stiff ties.

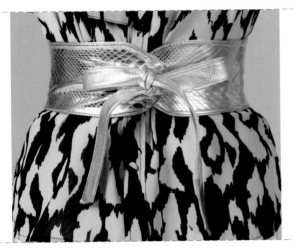

other must LOSE

- **Cummerbunds**
- **Wrap belts**
- **Corset belts**
- **Cinch belts**

sale suckers

It's not that obi-style belts aren't glamorous on the runway. These belts, which were inspired by the Japanese obi and first seen in the 1980s, are quite chic. But it's a tough style for most people to wear. It is truly meant for straight up-and-down body types with long, narrow torsos and no hips.

behind the seams

A feature of the Western obi-style belt is a thick tie at the front (in most traditional Japanese styles, the tie is in the back), which draws considerable attention to the stomach.

ditch it

I warn fellow short-waisted women that this is not a look for you. As a professional Japanese classical dancer, I wear obis with kimonos and find my chest resting atop the obi. The much-needed space between the waist and upper torso disappears. You don't want this to happen.

A medium-width strap with a rhinestone or crystal adornment that's proportional to the belt's width.

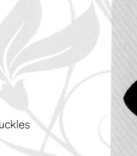

other must HAVES

+ **Glitter belts**
+ **Belts with grommets**
+ **Western belts** with statement buckles
+ **Paillette belts**

MATCH POINT

If you are belt shy, a belt in tune with an outfit's color scheme is an easy update that can bring the *right* amount of attention to your waist-line. After you're comfortable wearing belts, you can delve into delicately embellished styles for a touch of drama.

SHAPE SAVER

If you have hips, an embellished belt is a **save-me**. Wear this cincher at the waist to draw eyes to the upper body and away from the problem area. For an impressive array of designer belts you can search by category (designer, hip, skinny, waist), color, size, price, popularity, and newness, try Bluefly (www.bluefly.com).

AGE ALERT

Attention pregnant women: Since belts offer definition and accent to shapeless tunics, straight shifts, and oversized shirts, they can similarly offer style to a maternity wardrobe. Simply belt above or below the bump with a more generous belt size than you'd normally wear, and buckle to comfort—not constriction.

t.oss

An excessively studded rhinestone belt
with a super-sized buckle, in a hideous color.

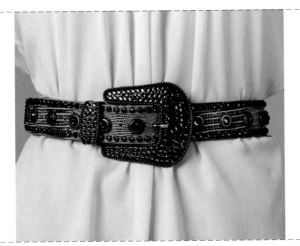

other must LOSE

- Rainbow **striped ribbon belts** from the '70s
- **Thickly braided belts**
- **Belts with huge bows**
- **Overly studded double buckle belts**

ditch it

Rhinestones done wrong are hideous: the glaring mix of shine and stud is blinding. Generally, if the rhinestones outshine anything else you are wearing, don't even think twice—just take the bling off.

raising the bar

I'm generally not a fan of rhinestones paired with any other embellishment. Think simple. A leather strap with a few studded rhinestones plus a monochromatic outfit? That's called rockin' the hardware.

age alert

The oversized logos on belt buckles are way too heavy metal—and I don't recommend them even if you're young. Why brand yourself with someone else's monogram? Your own initials, done right, can be cool though.

behind the seams

Beware of poor workmanship on a belt: Frayed threads along the edges, a too small or too large belt tongue that doesn't fit the holes, a buckle that quickly wears down the belt's material, and a strap that's stiff and doesn't conform to the shape of your body.

accessory box:
jewelry

Jewelry follows the Law of Attraction: Stand near a stunning piece and you'll want to look at it, touch it, have it! Given its shine and sparkle, jewelry can be the first thing we notice on a person. If I'm stumped on a clothes shopping mission but I find a few small pieces of jewelry (real or faux) to spruce up an existing outfit, I feel enormously successful.

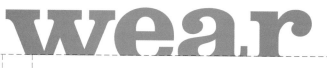

wear

Stud earrings in a round, square, or pear-shaped cut that reflects light from the stones.

other must HAVES

+ **Pearl studs**
+ **Diamond studs**
+ **Gold and silver studs** in unique designs
+ **Birthstone studs**

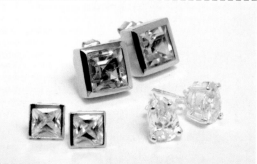

SHINING MOMENT

Stud shop at a store first rather than on the Internet. Studs don't photograph glamorously, so their finer selling points are difficult to view (that's why studs are rarely featured in fashion magazine spreads). Hold various shapes, colors, and metals to your lobes to see what speaks to them.

MATCH POINT

Studs serve smaller faces best. On a big face like mine, they just get lost. Given my large head and shocking volume of hair, I only wear studs to complement a larger necklace.

BEST BETS

Consider fresh options from Fragments, a New York jewelry store with multiple designers and price points (www.fragments.com), or Edition by Banana Republic, the brand's seasonally themed and location-inspired jewelry and accessories collection (www.bananarepublic.gap.com). New Twist (www.newtwist.com) has beautiful boho pieces.

ever wonder if you should test pearls against your teeth?

When rubbed against each other or against your teeth, real pearls should feel slightly gritty while fake pearls will feel smooth and slip right off. If in doubt, get the professional opinion of a gemologist.

IT'S A STEAL

For handcrafted, artisan jewelry at wholesale prices, including an extensive array of studs, check out www.etsy.com. For playful, petite designs, check out the incredibly affordable jewelry designer Carolee at www.carolee.com, available in most department stores. Don't miss designer collaborations like Anna Sheffield and Hollywood Intuition by Jaye Hersh for Target, www.target.com. And www.alltherageonline. com is a jewelry lover's paradise, with nothing over $50.

wear

Chandelier earrings that are jeweled,
dangly, and sparkly.

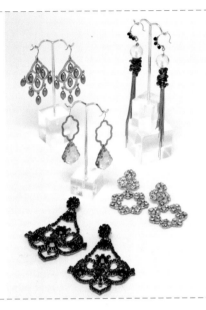

other must HAVES

+ **Hoops**
+ **Dressy crystal chandeliers** for evening; bohemian chandeliers in different materials for play
+ Solid, filigree or metallic **chandeliers for casual wear**
+ **Drop chain earrings**

SHINING MOMENT

Dangling chandelier earrings bring instant grace to any ensemble, casual or formal. They scream "sexy! sophisticated!" as they frame your face. These **save-me** earrings complement an array of face shapes: round, oval, heart, square. Only long faces should avoid chandelier earrings because they further lengthen.

RAISING THE BAR

It's essential to assess how a dangling earring looks in proportion to your head size and face. Danglers that hit your shoulder rarely work—the same goes for earrings so huge that they overwhelm a smaller face.

Divide chandeliers into small, medium, and long lengths, hold each one to your earlobe, and move a little in front of the mirror. Determine the size that flatters your proportions *the most,* and stick with that length.

IT'S A STEAL

Model turned actress Molly Sims has a lovely line of vintage-inspired jewelry called Grayce on HSN, which includes drop earrings, lariat necklaces, and layered link bracelets at great prices. For gorgeous fine jewelry, check out former Harry Winston guru Carol Brodie's new Rarities collection at the same site, www.hsn.com > jewelry.

AGE ALERT

If you are sensitive about the appearance of your neck, keep in mind that chandelier earrings bring attention to that area, from your collarbone to your jaw line. Unless you're wearing a high-neck top, try a medium-bodied earring or stud instead.

CHANDELIER EARRINGS

accessory box : jewelry

123

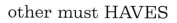
Wow-factor necklaces—some short, some long—loaded with embellishment, gems, and serious shine factor.

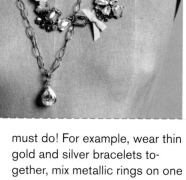

other must HAVES

+ **Single pendant necklaces**
+ **Bib necklaces**
+ **Personalized necklaces** (Three Sisters Jewelry, Laura James Jewelry, and Tina Tang Jewelry)

SHINING MOMENT

Wear a statement necklace with monochromatic clothes that have a simple neckline: think crew, V-neck, or bateau (boat-neck). A raucous print or an elaborate cut will detract from the attention the necklace brings to itself…and your face.

BEST BETS

Max & Chloe is a hot little store for one-stop jewelry shopping and features a number of boutique designs, including chandelier earrings by Ben-Amun and inexpensive gemmed pieces by

Calico Juno. A shop-by-price feature allows you to see what's $50 and $99 and under at a glance. www.maxandchloe.com

RAISING THE BAR

If you have a round face, it's best not to wear a heavy, round necklace that emphasizes that fact. A super weighty necklace may also overpower your neck. Consider a more delicate or longer style that will better suit you.

MATCH POINT

Mixing metals like gold, silver, and bronze is not only completely acceptable, it's the new

must do! For example, wear thin gold and silver bracelets together, mix metallic rings on one hand or wear a braided chain necklace of gold and bronze.

style to go

For jewelry with true inspirational meaning, get yoga-inspired jewelry from www.satyajewelry.com, and inscribed necklaces from www.givingtreejewelry.com and www.moondancejewelry.com.

toss

A very tight choker necklace with a dangling pendant that adds bulk to the neck.

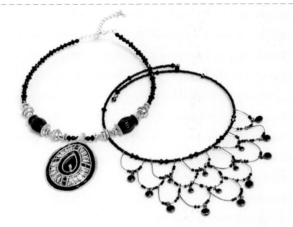

other must LOSE

- Velvet necklaces
- Dog collar-style chokers
- Heavily beaded chokers
- Ribbon or string-tied necklaces

ditch it

There is little that is redeeming about a choker, but I'm biased as a girl with a short neck. When worn incorrectly it enhances a double chin, slices the length of your neck in half, and seemingly cuts off your circulation.

match point

The choker is difficult to pair with the right clothes. Too much exposed décolletage and the choker feels lonely at the base of the neck. No extravagant, competing neck-lines, or this necklace will indeed choke your style.

best bets

Chokers seem to perform best with formal gowns—probably because when loaded with diamonds and gems, what's not to like? (Nicole Miller has tons of affordable options with glitz, www.nicolemiller.com). But I've never been a fan of the choker *with* matching earrings—simply too over the top unless the dress code is black tie.

it's a steal

The jewelry-exclusive site www.shopthelook.net has *extremely* affordable accessories with an impressive get-the-celeb-look-for-less homepage.

sale suckers

Whenever I'm on a beach vacation, I can't resist buying glass jewelry or hemp braided necklaces and hand-beaded pieces. Inevitably however, the shells chip and the hemp frays, and I rarely get wear beyond that trip. Sure, buy local, but be mindful that your trinket may only live on in photographs.

wear

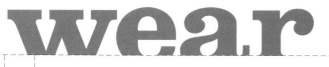

Bangle bracelets in a variety of materials, which can be worn alone or together to make a statement.

other must HAVES

+ **Statement cuffs**
+ Multiple strand **thin bangles and bracelets**
+ **Charm bracelets**

SHINING MOMENT

Welcome to the bangle revolution! Hammered to smooth metals, heavily embellished, and even coiled snakes have walked the runway and crept up our wrists. The bangle is a strong piece that exudes power, and it can be worn to complement nearly every other type of jewelry, thus making it a **save-me**.

INSOURCING

Whether you have bony or thick wrists, make sure your bangle—which is fixed in size—fits before you walk out of the store. Too big on thin wrists and your hands will look miniscule. Too tight on fuller wrists and you unattractively subdivide the arm. Cuffs are adjustable, so make sure you size to fit with a hint of wiggle room.

RAISING THE BAR

Bangles in resin, plastic, wood, acetate, faux bone, and bamboo are fun to wear individually but even more playful when stacked—as long as your co-workers are cool with the clanging. Pick a color or print from your ensemble to highlight.

BEST BETS

For bracelets (and necklaces) with body and substance, try J.Crew (www.jcrew.com).

toss

A single chain bracelet with a large, unattractive clasp and thin links that hangs limply from the wrist.

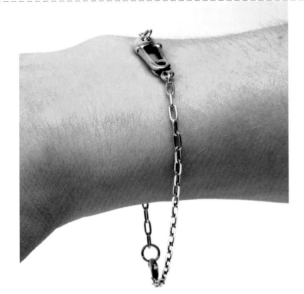

other must LOSE

- Chipped **shell bracelets**
- **Frayed friendship bracelets**
- **Bent wire bracelets**

ditch it

You might think a thin chain bracelet offers simple elegance, but in my opinion it gets lost on the wrist. In the '80s, my first gold snake chain bracelet constantly snagged on sweaters and bent itself into permanent kinks. So *if* you insist on this style, go for box, rolo, or mesh chains that offer a smoother look.

match point

Which metal complements your skin tone best? Turn your wrist over and look at the color of your veins. If they're green, you gravitate toward the warm color family of sunset hues like orange, red, and yellow; gold is your ideal match. If they're blue, you are in the cool color family of ocean hues like blue, purple, green; silver is your choice metal.

raising the bar

The way to make this teeny, tiny thin bracelet work is to pair it with other thin to medium bracelets and stack them along your wrist. Mix styles for a funky, offbeat look, like you've gone to four flea markets and purchased and layered a bracelet from each one. For pre-assembled thin bracelets, try Bee Charming at www.bcharming. net and check out their Leather Charm, Rubber, Piano Wire, and Million Beads collections.

wear

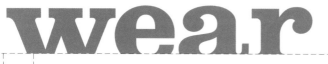

A delicate dress watch with a classic dial and either a leather or link-metal band.

other must HAVES

+ **Men's watches** that fit your wrist
+ **Colorful leather banded watches**
+ **Period pieces**, such as Art deco–inspired, '80s-inspired digital, vintage

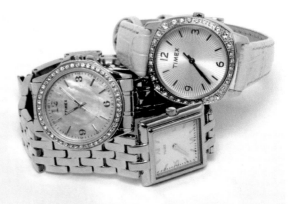

SHINING MOMENT

Most of us have at least one watch that we wear for every occasion. Up your arsenal with different timepieces for different looks. For a power suit, wear an oversized dial or a gold or silver dress watch. For evening, a crystal or diamond watch with mother-of-pearl inlay is perfect.

RAISING THE BAR

Own at least one watch with a leather strap and another watch with a link band. A link watch doubles as a bracelet, while leather bands bridge both casual and dressy demands.

BEST BETS

Women wearing men's watches is a growing trend. Whether you like a more substantial, broader faced watch or wear it as a power move, make sure the band fits. Poke holes in a leather band. Remove links in a metal band—many watches allow you to do this without additional tools. If not, take it to a watch shop for a quick fix.

IT'S A STEAL

Timex is my go-to brand for exquisite, everyday watches. As a spokesperson, I know that, for unbeatable prices, you'll get stunning variety, functions, and value. Timex's Women's T-series Chronograph or Sport Luxury series offers oversized designs with a woman in mind, for sporty functionality that works from day to night. In recent years, exclusive design and distribution deals with J. Crew, Bloomingdales, and Barneys New York have upped the ante. Check out the buzz and my blog at www.timexstylewatch.com.

style to go

When selecting a men's watch for yourself, make sure the larger size dial (the face) does not exceed the width of your wrist.

A black, canvas, or plastic-banded digital sports watch of shoddy workmanship.

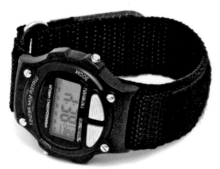

other must LOSE

- **Watches with fraying straps or chipped metal bands**

- **Timepieces that don't keep accurate time**

- **Watches with irreparably scratched faces**, unless they have sentimental value (Grandpa's military watch)

ditch it

Sports watches (usually digital, with chronograph, timer, alarm functions, heart rate monitor, etc.) are ideal for active and leisure activities, but up the style quotient with dress casual and formal watches for everything else. A traditional sports watch is an eyesore when paired with a polished suit.

sale suckers

Don't be charmed into buying a cheap ticker of poor quality that will tarnish and leave a black ring on your wrist. Check the metal of the band (yes to stainless steel, no to nickel plating or worse), the quality of the strap (genuine leather as opposed to flimsy plastic), and the brand's reputation. Resist street vendors.

insourcing

It takes a mere $5 to have a watch battery changed, and it's free if you have the tools to easily do it yourself. Don't be lazy and buy a quick-fix watch just because your other watches stopped ticking.

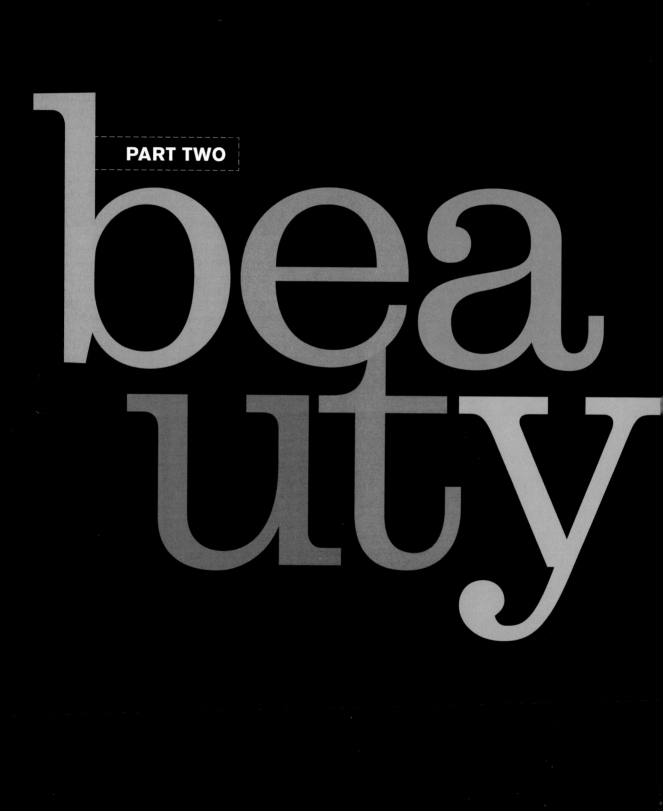

PART TWO

beauty

I have beauty editor friends whose desks, bins, and offices overflow with the latest high-end products—some of which are still in lab-testing tubs. I have other friends who, late for whatever they're doing that day, realize while looking in the car's rearview mirror that they forgot to even wash their face, much less put on mascara.

Then there is the general reporter like me who is fascinated by both the technology of prestige products and the affordability of miracle-working mass brands. I unabashedly mix things up. I'm the consummate tester of everything beauty and right now my dining room table resembles a cosmetics emporium. My friends have been coming over to visit—and it's not to see me!

For this section, I get to fling on the hat of a full-fledged beauty editor. We'll go to your beauty shelves and drawers and apply the same Wear This, Toss That! inventory gusto to skincare (Chapter 8), makeup (Chapter 9), and haircare (Chapter 10) that we did to fashion. I have lots of info for everyone—even for those who don't wear a drop of makeup (see Natural vs. Naked, pages 166–167). I call upon my favorite experts to give us their best techniques and answer long-standing beauty questions that both you and I have—like when do I start using a serum, how do I find the right shade of red lipstick, and should I stress about sulfates in shampoos?

I've tested all the items here. My husband says I have the perfect skin for this, because it's sensitive. I've had the itches, the rashes, and the occasional adverse reaction (in addition to disappointment with products that didn't deliver), all in the name of finding top performers that will save you money and keep you looking sensational.

You should know that mass-market brands invest just as much money in research, marketing, and development as prestige brands do, because everyone wants your business. With that in mind, I include both ends of the price spectrum, and often a mid-range. You'll find:

THE DEAL ($): grab-and-go steals you can buy without guilt.

LITTLE LUXURY ($$): slight splurges that are worthy small investments because they work.

THE ULTIMATE ($$$): wish list items that we pray others gift us!

Think of these pricing categories as a general guide, designed with a particular product's price range in mind. For example, I consider both a 99-cent lip liner and an $11 foundation The Deal purchases because they are at the low-cost end of their product categories. (And in Chapter 9 look for "The Natural," which are products that attempt a purer approach.) Throughout these beauty pages, you'll find high-per-

skincare shelf

cleansing, moisturizing, anti-aging & preventive, body care

cleansing

cleansers

THE DEAL $

Aveeno Positively Radiant Cleanser, $7; drugstores and other mass retailers

THE LITTLE LUXURY $$

Shiseido The Skincare Extra Gentle Cleansing Foam, $28; Macy's or www.sca.shiseido.com for stores

THE ULTIMATE $$$

The Organic Pharmacy's Carrot Butter Cleanser, $59.95; www.theorganicpharmacy.com

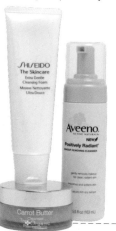

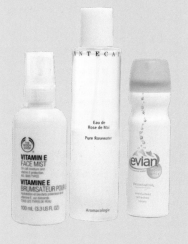

mists

THE DEAL $

Evian Brumisateur Mineral Water Spray, $5.50; www.amazon.com

THE LITTLE LUXURY $$

The Body Shop Vitamin E Face Mist, $16; www.thebodyshop-usa.com

THE ULTIMATE $$$

Chantecaille Pure Rosewater, $55; www.chantecaille.com

facial exfoliators

THE DEAL $

Neutrogena Deep Clean Gentle Scrub, $6.49, or Neutrogena Deep Clean Relaxing Nightly Scrub, $7.49; www.neutrogena.com

St. Ives Timeless Skin Daily Microdermabrasion, $4.99; drugstores and other mass retailers

THE LITTLE LUXURY $$

Nude Skincare Facial Scrub, $52; www.nudeskincare.com

THE ULTIMATE $$$

Dr. Brandt Microdermabrasion Exfoliating Face Cream, $75; www.drbrandtskincare.com

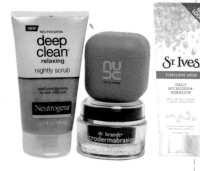

BEST BETS

Speaking as a working woman and a mom, who has *time* for multiple steps when it comes to cleaning *anything*? The Organic Pharmacy—a new and fabulous organic products online store (www.theorganicpharmacy.com)—has a cult-following Carrot Butter Cleanser that is worth every counter-intuitive step: massage a dime-size amount onto a dry, dirty, made-up face, allow to sit, then wipe off gently with a warm washcloth. Result?

A clean face that feels so soft you *may* skip moisturizing!

APPLY THIS

When it comes to sloughing off dead skin cells, how do we measure up with the rest of the world? "Americans don't exfoliate enough, and when they do, they tend to use the wrong products," says Kate Somerville, aesthetician to stars like Eva Mendes and Kate Walsh. In a nutshell…avoid certain products. "Don't pick scrubs made

from crushed nuts and seeds, which are jagged and irritate the skin. Look for round beads and enzymes," says Somerville. She recommends ExfoliKate Intensive Exfoliating Treatment ($85, www.katesomerville.com). "It's a one-of-a-kind product combining enzymes, gentle acids, and microbeads for multi-dimensional exfoliation."

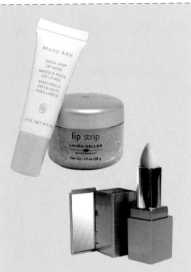

lip exfoliators

THE DEAL $

Mary Kay Satin Lips Lip Mask, $9.50; www.marykay.com

THE LITTLE LUXURY $$

Tarte FRXtion Lip Balm, $15; www.tartecosmetics.com

THE ULTIMATE $$$

Laura Geller Lip Strip, $19; www.laurageller.com

other must HAVES

+ **To-go cleansing wipes:** Garnier Nutritioniste Nutri-Pure Oil-free Dextoxifying Wet Cleaning Towelettes, $5.99; drugstores and other mass retailers; or Josie Maran's Bare Naked Wipes, $12; www.josiemaran.com

+ Gentle **eye makeup remover:** Lancome Bi-Facil Double-Action Eye Makeup Remover, $26; www.lancome-usa.com; or Bare Escentuals i.d. bareEyes Eye Makeup Remover, $14; www.bareescentuals.com, www.ulta.com

THE SCOOP

Is toner (a.k.a. astringent) necessary? There's controversy among dermatologists, aestheticians, and beauty editors. In the past, cleansers weren't as effective as they are now, so women felt the need to clean further with a toner—and an additional skincare step was born. But today's cleansers are highly efficient at removing impurities, and a toner often over-dries your skin. In the Mists category, I list my favorite mists and atomizers, which are the gentler hydrating cousins of the toner, to satisfy those who wish to feel refreshed without the dehydration.

STRIPPING DOWN: UNCOVERING EXFOLIATION!

From celebrity aesthetician Kate Somerville

NORMAL SKIN

Even flawless skin has dead skin cells on the surface, making skin look dull. Exfoliate, and young, healthy cells resurface, so skin appears smooth and beautiful. Use a gentle exfoliator with enzymes, gentle acids, and microbeads.

DRY SKIN

Exfoliation is essential with dry skin, as dead cells pile up on the skin's surface. Exfoliation also keeps pores clear of debris and makes them appear smaller.

OILY SKIN

If you're prone to breakouts, you still need to exfoliate, but gently. Select a chemical exfoliant with salicylic acid that won't scrub at the blemishes on the surface and cause irritation.

HOW OFTEN

If you have healthy skin, exfoliate twice a week; sensitive or more mature skin, once a week.

moisturizing

day moisturizers

THE DEAL $

Olay Active Hydrating Beauty Fluid Original, $7.29; drugstores and other mass retailers

THE LITTLE LUXURY $$

Josie Maran Argan Oil, $48, or Argan Oil Moisturizing Stick, $22; www.josiemaran.com

THE ULTIMATE $$$

Nude Skincare Age Defense Intense Moisturizer, $100; www.nudeskincare.com

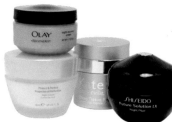

night moisturizers

THE DEAL $

Boots No7 Protect and Perfect Night Cream, $19.99; Target stores or www.target.com

THE LITTLE LUXURY $$

Olay Regenerist Continuous Night Recovery Moisturizing Treatment, $21; drugstores and other mass retailers

THE ULTIMATE $$$

Kate Somerville Deep Tissue Repair Cream with Peptide K8, $150; www.katesomerville.com

Shiseido Future Solution LX Total Revitalizing Cream, $260; Nordstrom or www.sca.shiseido.com for stores

eye creams

THE DEAL $

RoC Multi-Correxion Eye Treatment, $24.99; drugstores and other mass retailers

THE LITTLE LUXURY $$

Borba Orbital Eye Rejuvenator, $38; www.borba.com

THE ULTIMATE $$$

Kinerase Pro+ Therapy Ultra Rich Eye Repair, $88; www.kinerase.com

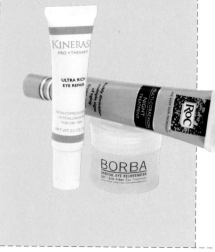

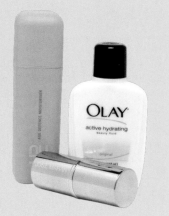

THE SCOOP

My secret sunscreen hails from Japan: Bioré UV Perfect Face Milk. It goes on silky, turns matte, and works like a makeup primer; and it doesn't stick or stink, the way so many sunscreens do. All my friends love it. I should become a distributor.

BEST BETS

As a day/night moisturizer, Shiseido Bio-Performance Super Restoring Cream ($98) has been my **save-me** for years.

That is, until Shiseido created a new line, Future Solution LX (I love the nighttime Total Revitalizing Cream), which gives skin newborn softness. How does it work? Through an innovative technology called Skingencell 1P, which promotes the growth of strong, healthy cells. Since I'm allergic to a number of designer moisturizers at comparable price points, this is my new splurge. It's decadent, so you can use it sparingly. As with most Shiseido products, it's lightly scented.

IT'S A STEAL

I'm obsessed with eye creams because the eyes are one of the first places we see fine lines and wrinkles. RoC is a French skincare brand that was the first to formulate and package retinol, or pure vitamin A—the anti-aging wonder that helps skin regenerate and combat signs of aging. Within weeks, their Multi-Correxion Eye Treatment reduces the appearance of wrinkles, dark circles, and puffiness. As with all retinol

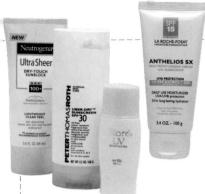

sunscreens, face

THE DEAL $

Neutrogena Ultra Sheer Dry Touch Sunblock, SPF 55, 70, 85, $10.99; www.drugstore.com

THE LITTLE LUXURY $$

Bioré UV Perfect Face Milk, SPF 50+ PA+++ in white, $15; www.bonanzle.com or www.ebay.com

Peter Thomas Roth Uber Dry Sunscreen SPF 30, $26; www.peterthomasroth.com

THE ULTIMATE $$$

La Roche-Posay Anthelios Daily Moisturizing Cream SPF 15, $29; www.laroche-posay.us

ever wonder what those little white bumps are around your eyes?

They are called milia and are caused by using too heavy an eye cream, which smothers the thin skin around the eyes. "That's why you need an eye cream labeled as both non-comedogenic as well as ophthalmologist approved," says DERMAdoctor founder Dr. Audrey Kunin. Milia are difficult to remove by yourself, so have your dermatologist "pick" them open with a sterile lancet and curette them off.

other must HAVES

+ Moisturizing **lip balm with SPF** (see Lip Balm: A Smackers Smackdown!, page 143)

+ **Eye gel** for de-puffing and for oily skin types

+ **Body sunscreen**: DERMAdoctor Body Guard Exquisitely Light SPF 30 for face and body, $25; www.dermadoctor.com or 1-877-DERMADR

MOISTURIZING

skincare shelf

products, dive in slowly and use sparingly, as they are potent and can cause irritation.

TRICKS OF THE TRADE

Argan oil, made from the nut of a tree that hails from southwestern Morocco, is rich in the antioxidant vitamin E and fatty acids. It's all the rage now because it mimics the natural oil environment of the skin *and* has anti-aging properties. In

her new makeup and skincare line, Josie Maran, former cover model turned cosmetic entrepreneur with a conscience, has infused most of her products with this miracle substance. Her 100 Percent Argan Oil can be used as a day and night moisturizer, and the Argan Oil Moisturizing Stick is great for all other dry body parts in need of rescue. www.josiemaran.com

BEST BETS

Wonder how pure and effective "natural" skincare really is? Allow the UK-import Nude, a natural skincare company, to strip away impure thoughts. Nude uses pre- and probiotics to deliver products that pass impressive muster in clinical trials. In addition to saturating skin with moisture, Nude's Age Defense Moisturizer reduces the appearance of wrinkles by 65 percent (www.nudeskincare.com) and I love the unusual orchid scent.

masks

THE DEAL $

MD Formulations Moisture Defense Antioxidant Treatment Masque, $26; www.bareescentuals.com

THE LITTLE LUXURY $$

Estée Lauder Resilience Lift Extreme Ultra Firma Mask, $40; www.esteelauder.com

THE ULTIMATE $$$

Nude Skincare Miracle Mask, $62; www.nudeskincare.com

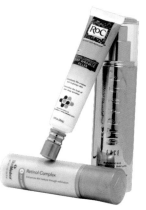

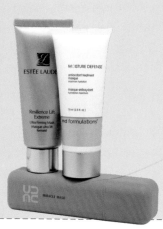

spot treatments

THE DEAL $

RoC Retinol Correxion Deep Wrinkle Filler, $21.95; drugstores and other mass retailers

THE LITTLE LUXURY $$

SkinMedica Age Defense Retinol Complex, $53; www.skinmedica.com

THE ULTIMATE $$$

Elizabeth Arden's Prevage Face Advanced Anti-aging Serum, $155; www.prevageskin.com

serums

THE DEAL $

Lumene Excellent Future Deep Repairing Serum, $29.99; drugstores and other mass retailers

THE LITTLE LUXURY $$

Kate Somerville Quench Hydrating Face Serum, $65; www.katesomerville.com

THE ULTIMATE $$$

Estée Lauder Perfectionist (CP+) Wrinkle Lifting Serum, $80; www.esteelauder.com

Shiseido Bio-Performance Super Corrective Serum, $80; Lord & Taylor or www.sca.shiseido.com for stores

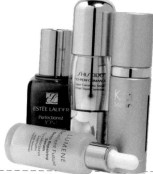

THE SCOOP

Serums (applied after you wash your face and before you moisturize) are designed to deliver vital nutrients deeper into the skin cells to hydrate, plump, and nourish. While a scrub physically removes dead cells, a serum quietly encourages skin cell resurfacing. "Start using a serum in your late 20s," advises Kate Somerville, creator and director of Kate Somerville Skin Health Experts. Apply morning and night, and seal the serum with a moisturizer. Remember, says Somerville, it should feel lightweight and absorb readily without feeling sticky or clogging pores.

TRICKS OF THE TRADE

Elizabeth Arden's new Prevage Face Advance Anti-aging Serum (www.prevageskin.com) is a technologically advanced formulation, binding idebenone, one of the most powerful antioxidants available without a prescription, with a lipid so that it is stored and used in a natural, time-release method—when the skin needs it. In a clinical trial, testers saw a 75 percent reduction in fine lines and wrinkles after eight weeks. It can reduce the appearance of minor scars, too.

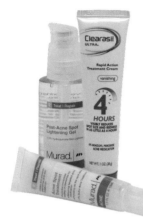

acne treatment creams

THE DEAL $
New Clearasil Ultra Rapid Action Treatment Cream, $9.99; www.drugstore.com

THE LITTLE LUXURY $$
Murad Acne Spot Treatment, $18; www.murad.com

THE ULTIMATE $$$
Murad Post-Acne Spot Lightening Gel, $60; www.murad.com

86 percentage of women who use a makeup product with skincare benefits

other must HAVES

+ Body spot treatment cream that reverses sun damage, diminishing the appearance of age spots: Nia24 Sun Damage Repair for Décolletage and Hands, $55; www.nia24.com

+ Knock-out-the-wrinkles **neck cream**: Dr. Brandt Time Arrest V-Zone Neck Cream, $60; www.drbrandtskincare.com

+ Dark circle diminisher: Murad Lighten and Brighten Eye Treatment uses hydroquinone to lighten under-eye circles by up to 59 percent, $67; www.murad.com

skincare shelf

AGE ALERT
"While moisturizers, anti-aging creams, and sunscreens are lathered carefully on the face and body, the neck skin is neglected," says celebrity dermatologist Dr. Fredric Brandt. The result? "Skin can become wrinkled, loose, and crepey in texture." Dr. Brandt's Time Arrest V-Zone Neck Cream (www.drbrandtskincare.com) works like the skin's GPS, carrying glycolic acid and vitamin C into the deepest layers of the epidermis, targeting problem areas to repair and restore skin's structure."

BEST BETS
Nia24 Skin Strengthening Complex ($85; www.nia24.com) is an overall anti-aging moisturizer that uses 5 percent topical niacin to strengthen skin from within, actually reversing the effects of sun damage. I put this product to the test to see if it reduced the numerous sunspots that appeared during my pregnancy (when increased facial pigmentation is common). In clinical trials, hyperpigmentation was reduced by 90 percent, and sure enough after four weeks of use, I saw a dramatic lightening of my spots.

from the mouths of mavens: **SCOTT-VINCENT BORBA**

I met Licensed Esthetician and Makeup Artist, Nutraceutical Specialist and TV personality Scott-Vincent Borba (fans include Megan Fox, Jennifer Love Hewitt, Selena Gomez, and Jane Krakowski) at the opening of CVS's flagship Beauty 360 store in Washington, D.C. He's the founder of Borba skincare and co-founder of e.l.f. (Eyes Lips Face) Cosmetics, and he previously worked in research and development for companies such as Neutrogena, Sebastian, Proctor & Gamble, Joico, Hard Candy, and Shiseido. Scott-Vincent brings a unique approach to his namesake line of nutraceuticals (nourishing healthy skin from the inside out) and cosmeceuticals (topical applications). He also shares some table-turning ideas on how to approach our daily beauty rituals regarding toner, exfoliation, and eye creams.

What are your feelings about toner? Is it a necessary step in the beauty routine?

Toner should be eradicated. It was created as an old-school solution twenty years ago to extract oil from the dermis, leaving skin feeling clean and minimizing pores, but it really has the reverse effect.

For the average person, toners, many of which contain alcohol, remove too much oil, robbing skin of the natural oil it needs for healthy hydration. This over-dries the skin and causes an overproduction of sebum in the glands, which can clog pores and lead to acne. An increased acneaic environment actually reveals more lines and wrinkles. That said, 70 percent of consumers still want and use toner!

If toner is a no go, then what's the answer?

Finding the right cleanser and serum combination that hydrates the skin without using toner. The consumer, however, craves that liquid feeling and cleansing action, so I make all of my products multitaskers. My Age Defying 4-in-1 Cleansing Treatment is a cleanser, pore refiner, makup remover, and microdermabrasion all in one. It starts as a foam, becomes a liquid, and then finishes with microdermabrasion.

How does the average woman perform when it comes to exfoliation?

Most Americans are under-exfoliating.

How often should we exfoliate?

The real issue has more to do with when we do it in our routine and not how often. Most people cleanse, then exfoliate. Let's say your cleanser has beneficial hydrating properties, as so many do. If you exfoliate after cleansing you strip the skin of these benefits.

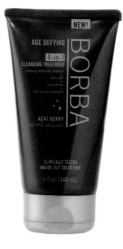

And your exfoliation approach?

My approach is radically different from what I learned in aesthetician school, from what doctors will tell you, and from everything you've ever heard. I suggest exfoliation followed by a non-abrasive cleanser. Most people usually do the opposite and cleanse first, which doesn't remove the free radicals, pollution, and sebum your dermis collects over the course of the day. You need to jackhammer that up from the get go with an exfoliation followed by a gentle cleanser.

What do you look for in an exfoliator?

That the exfoliator is spherical or round, like those I use in my micro diamonds, jojoba beads, and argan oil. If it's jagged in shape like you find in so many brands that use walnuts or apricots, you literally overly microabrade the skin, allowing free radicals to penetrate the first and second layers of the dermis, which leads to more aging, bacterial growth, and acne.

I'm a fanatic about eye creams.

In my research, women as young as 18 years old suffer from a crepey eyelid that makes them look not well rested. But because the upper lid is the thinnest area of skin of the entire body, most eye creams cannot be applied there…they can be irritating or burning. So I developed the Orbital Eye Rejuvenator and named it "orbital" for a precise reason: You can use the mousse-like cream both below and above the eye. Apply the cream below the eye and by the time you apply it to the upper lid—from the temple to the inner socket area—your undereye will be de-puffed. It works like an eye shadow primer for the upper lid and an eye cream simultaneously, and so it's a two-in-one product.

Where do we err when it comes to eye creams?

The average woman uses concealer with the intent of locking in moisture, but it's not good enough. Use an eye cream twice a day. If anything, you need to attack this area to look ageless because it is the first place where signs of aging, like fine lines and wrinkles, are evident.

70
percentage of what you put on your skin that is absorbed into your bloodstream

skincare shelf

body care

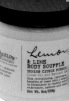

skincare shelf

BODY CARE

body soaps & washes

THE DEAL $

Dove Beauty Bar, $2.99 for three bars; drugstores and other mass retailers

THE LITTLE LUXURY $$

AHAVA Mineral Botanic, cream body washes, $21.50; Ulta Beauty www.ulta.com or www.ahavaus.com

Fresh Sugar Lemon Shower Gel, $18.50; www.fresh.com

THE ULTIMATE $$$

Clarins Relax Bath & Shower Concentrate, $27.50; www.usclarins.com

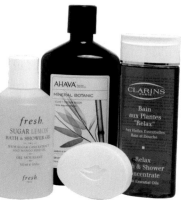

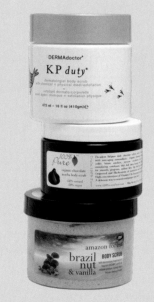

body exfoliators

THE DEAL $

Boots Amazon Forest Brazil Nut & Vanilla Body Scrub, $9.99; www.target.com or www.us.boots.com

THE LITTLE LUXURY $$

100 Percent Pure Organic Body Scrub, $22; www.100percentpure.com

DERMAdoctor KP Duty dermatologist body scrub with chemical + physical medi-exfoliation, $44; www.dermadoctor.com

THE ULTIMATE $$$

REN Moroccan Rose Otto Sugar Body Polish, $60; www.renskincare.com

body lotions & butters

THE DEAL $

Cetaphil Daily Advance Ultra Hydrating Lotion, $9.99; drugstores and other mass retailers

THE LITTLE LUXURY $$

C.O. Bigelow Lemon & Lime Body Soufflé, $15; www.bigelow chemists.com

The Body Shop Body Butter, $20; www.thebodyshop-usa.com

THE ULTIMATE $$$

Elizabeth Arden Prevage Body Total Transforming Anti-aging Moisturizer, $135; www.prevage skin.com

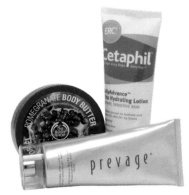

LIP BALM: A SMACKERS SMACKDOWN!

THE DEAL $

LypSyl LypMoisturizer Original Formula, $2.99; www.lypsylhome.com or www.walgreens.com

Burt's Bees Beeswax Lip Balm, $3; www.burtsbees.com or 800-849-7112

Chapstick Overnight Lip Treatment, $3.99; www.chapstick.com or www.drugstore.com

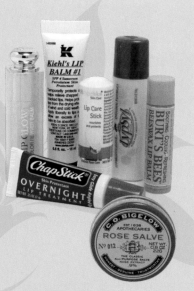

THE LITTLE LUXURY $$

C.O. Bigelow Rose Salve, $5.50; www.bigelowchemists.com or mass retailers

Kiehl's Lip Balm #1 with SPF 4, $7; www.kiehls.com

Dr. Hauschka Lip Care Stick, $13.95; www.drhauschka.com

THE ULTIMATE $$$

Dior Addict Lip Glow Color Reviver Balm with SPF 10, $28; www.dior.com or 866-503-9490; Neiman Marcus, www.neimanmarcus.com or 888-888-4757

other must HAVES

+ **Hand lotion** that deeply moisturizes without making hands slippery: ~H2O+ Hand and Nail Cream, $17; www.h2oplus.com or 800-242-2284

+ Targeted **hand and foot scrub** that gives you an instant, at-home spa treatment: Barielle 60-second Mani-Pedi, $25; www.barielle.com or 800-790-8884

+ **Complete body cream** that does it all (note that it has a strong medicinal scent): Japan's Yu-Be Moisturizing Skin Cream, $24; www.amazon.com or drugstores and other mass retailers

+ **An ointment for immediate relief of chapped lips**, Aquaphor Lip Repair, $4.99; www.aquaphorhealing.com

TRICKS OF THE TRADE

Like a chameleon, Dior Addict Lip Glow changes hue, adjusting to each woman's lip chemistry to enhance her natural lip color. It's also a premium moisturizer for your smackers. It contains wild mango, so watch out if you're allergic.

IT'S A STEAL

AHAVA's new cream body washes are free of harsh cleansers and are heavenly for sensitive skin types. The creams use natural plant and fruit extracts and the line's signature Dead Sea minerals. Lightly fragranced, the seven varieties (like Pansy & Bamboo and Honeysuckle & Lavender) leave skin ultra-soft after washing. Warning: If you love lather, use a loofah or sponge to generate suds. I like the Nylon Body Towel–Soft Type for $4.25 from Muji (www.muji.us).

THE SCOOP

Beware of two-in-one body washes that also contain moisturizer, unless you love washing your tub. The moisturizing agents may leave your skin soft, but will also leave a waxy ring of build-up around your bathtub in no time.

I've been wearing sunscreen on my face since I was 11 years old. Although I love the sun, work in the garden, and play at the beach, I equally fear the powerful damage it can inflict. (It's also a Japanese thing to seriously covet porcelain skin.)

How many of you are equally cautious? Are you wearing sunscreen right now? Since it's time for a sunscreen showdown, I didn't hesitate to ask dermatologist Dr. Audrey Kunin, president and founder of DERMAdoctor and creator of the hugely informative and award-winning web site www.dermadoctor.com, for her insights on what we all should know when it comes to protecting our skin from the sun's rays.

In a nutshell, Dr. Kunin, this is what I know.

- Look for full-spectrum sunscreens (which are chemical agents) or sunblocks (which are physical blockers) that block both UVA (aging) and UVB (burning) rays.

- SPF stands for "sun protection factor." Basically, on a person who would normally get a sunburn in ten minutes, an SPF 15 sunscreen will enable them to stay in the sun fifteen times longer—150 minutes before they burn.

- Wear a minimum of SPF 15 daily, but consider SPF 30 for more protection.

- Reapply sunscreen every two hours.

- Avoid PABA or Para Aminobenzoic Acid (a chemical that absorbs UVB rays) if you have sensitive skin, as it can be an irritant.

What am I missing?

That there's no such thing as a waterproof sunscreen. Regardless of the label, if you read the fine print you'll see that you need to reapply SPF after getting out of the water or after towel-drying. Plus, you still need to reapply every two hours. Unfortunately, many consumers become confused by the term "waterproof" and fail to follow these guidelines, leaving them exposed to potential ultraviolet damage.

Any other irritants we should be aware of?

Fragrance is the number one allergen found in anything applied to the skin. If you are experiencing a reaction, consider the fragrance and color in the product first.

Is it necessary to buy sunscreen formulated for the face? Or can a body sunscreen work doubly for the face?

Sunscreen is sunscreen. We tend to get caught up in marketing, but a non-comedogenic [doesn't clog the pores] sunscreen can be applied to the face as well as the body. No need to pay an up-charge to own two different products.

If our makeup contains SPF then do we need to supplement with additional sunscreen or not?

There are several reasons why an SPF in a makeup or moisturizer should be considered icing on the cake and not be the sole SPF protection one chooses. First of all, many women apply cosmetics unevenly or just in certain areas where they need them. This can leave areas of the face, as well as neck, décolletage, and backs of the hands vulnerable. Second, makeup tends to wear off more easily than an SPF base. Third, many makeup products contain an SPF below 15.

So no matter what, we need an SPF base.

Apply your SPF to your face and other exposed skin daily, as if you were headed to the beach. Then feel free to apply or reapply your makeup.

How about SPF in lip products?

The lips are so commonly overlooked when it comes to sun protection. Make sure you either choose a lip color that contains a minimum SPF of 15, or apply some form of balm or lip product that contains an SPF before applying your color.

Does this irritate the lips?

If you are sensitive to chemical sunscreens, try applying one that contains a physical blocker, such as zinc oxide or titanium dioxide.

What sunscreen products do you recommend?

For someone looking for a physical blocker, I love the selections from Total Block. They contain iron oxide that helps block UVC, which is important for anyone with a sun allergy or a sun-sensitive medical condition such as lupus.

And for lip sunscreen?

Total Block SPF 45 LipCotz is a physical blocking lip balm; I also like Vanicream Lip Protectant SPF 30 and Neutrogena Lip Moisturizer SPF 15.

skincare shelf

ever wonder why you have to wear sunscreen on a cloudy day at the beach?

Because 90 percent of the sun's UV rays pass right through clouds and sand reflects a surprising 25 percent. And beware of the highest UV hours: 10am-2pm.

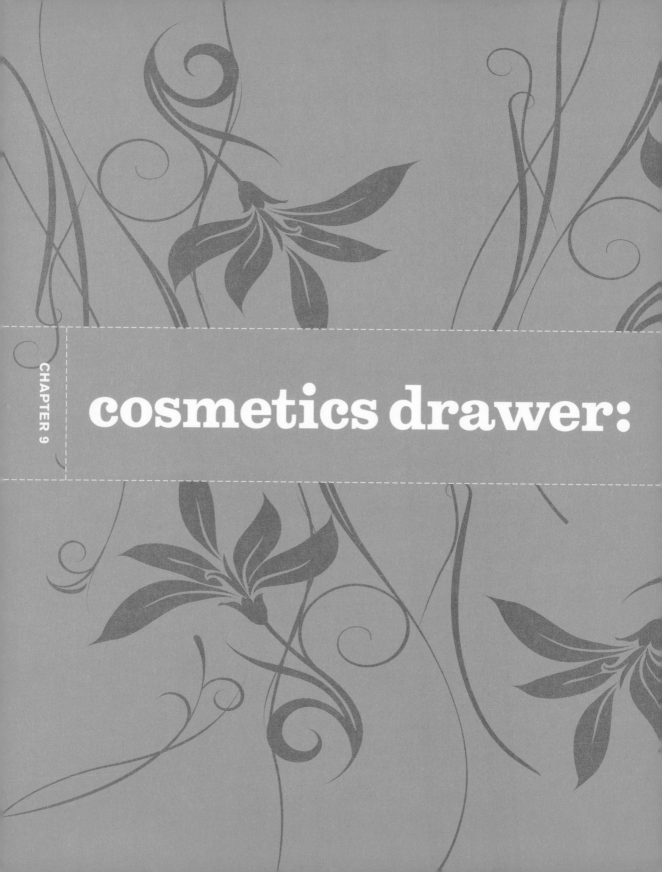

cosmetics drawer:

base, cheeks & brows, eyes, lips, tools

base

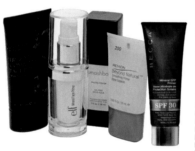

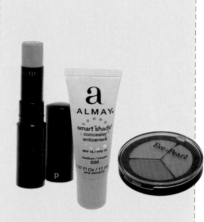

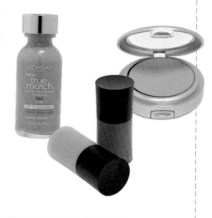

cosmetics drawer

BASE

makeup primers

THE DEAL $

e.l.f. Cosmetics Mineral Face Primer, $6; www.eyeslipsface.com

Revlon Beyond Natural Smoothing Primer, $12.99; www.revlon.com; drugstores and other mass retailers

THE ULTIMATE $$$

Global Goddess Upgrade Complexion Face Primer, $36; www.globalgoddessbeauty.com

Smashbox Photo Finish Foundation Primer, $36; www.smashbox.com or 888-763-1361

Becca Mineral SPF Primer SPF 30, $42; www.beccacosmetics.com

concealers

THE DEAL $

Almay SmartShade Concealer, $9; drugstores and other mass retailers

THE ULTIMATE $$$

Eve Pearl Concealer Trio, $50; www.evepearl.com

Cle de Peau Beauté Concealer (ivory, ocher, beige, honey), $70; www.cledepeau-beaute.com for stores or www.bergdorfgoodman.com

foundations

THE DEAL $

L'Oréal Paris True Match Super-Blendable Makeup, $10.95; drugstores and other mass retailers

THE ULTIMATE $$$

Giorgio Armani Beauty Lasting Silk UV Foundation, $58; Saks Fifth Avenue or www.giorgioarmanibeauty.com

THE NATURAL

4-in-1 Pressed Mineral Makeup SPF 15 by Pür Minerals, $25; Dillards or www.purminerals.com

---

TRICKS OF THE TRADE

A primer fills in imperfections and smoothes the face for makeup application. Primers also reduce shine on oily skin. It's an extra step, but it keeps your makeup looking fresh all day.

BEST BETS

Never use concealer? Neither did I...until I went on TV and realized it was miracle makeup. It brightens eyes *and* eliminates dark circles and puffiness. When I'm on *Today*, the makeup crew uses Eve Pearl's eponymous line of blendable concealers. Eve is an award-winning makeup artist and the talent behind Meredith Viera's beautifully made up face. Another brand I love is Bye Bye Under Eye by It Cosmetics because it's waterproof, $24; www.itcosmetics.com.

SPOTLIGHT ON HUE

Concealer should be one shade *lighter* than your facial skin tone. Foundation should *match* your facial skin tone. Always test on your face, not your wrist, arm, or hand, because skin can be a different color there. Seasons affect makeup shades, too. In summer, we need a darker concealer and foundation, and in winter, a lighter shade. Don't use one shade all year round unless your skin color truly stays the same. Makeup artist Leslie Marnett loves Revlon Custom Creations SPF 15 Foundation ($13.99; drugstores and other mass retailers). With its turn dial, the foundation can be adjusted to reflect the color of your skin.

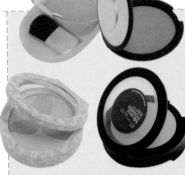

pressed powder cakes

THE DEAL $

CoverGirl TruBlend Pressed Powder, $8.47; drugstores and other mass retailers

Maybelline New York Mineral Power Finishing Veil Pressed Powder, $9.35; drugstores and other mass retailers

THE ULTIMATE $$$

Becca Fine Pressed Powder, $42; www.beccacosmetics.com

THE NATURAL

Physicians Formula Organic Wear Face Powder, $13.95; www.physiciansformula.com

loose powders

THE DEAL $

bareMinerals Original SPF15 Foundation ($25) and Mineral Veil ($19), www.ulta.com or www.bareescentuals.com

THE ULTIMATE $$$

Shu Uemura Face Powder Matte, $39, or Face Powder Sheer, $33; www.shuuemura-usa.com

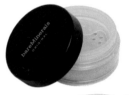

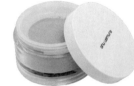

for women of color: top picks for darker skin tones

Black Opal True Color Crème Stick Foundation SPF 8 is a favorite of many makeup artists, $8.95; www.blackopalbeauty .com or drugstores and other mass retailers

Iman Cosmetics, an award-winning brand dedicated to products for women of color, www.imancosmetics.com

MAC Cosmetics, where diverse color options speak to diverse skin tones, www.maccosmetics.com

Becca Cosmetics, with thirty-four concealers and thirty foundation shades to choose from, www.beccacosmetics.com

APPLY THIS

Apply cream concealers with a synthetic brush (apply powder concealers with a natural bristle brush) beginning from the inner corner of the eye, across the lower eye to the outer eye corner—a half moon shape. Not an artist with the brushes? Gently warm the concealer between your thumb and ring finger before applying with the ring finger in a gentle, dabbing motion. I also dab concealer on other discolorations, like the pregnancy "wine stain" under my nose that never went away. Hot tip: Apply to the inner corner of your upper eyelid to make eyes pop.

DITCH IT

Remember: Nothing makes you look more like a novice than a demarcation of foundation that hangs like a cliff on the end of your chin. If you see a dividing line of color *anywhere* on your face, you need to blend—and most likely find makeup that's better matched to your skin tone.

IT'S A STEAL

It's nearly impossible to determine which shade of foundation is right for your skin at the drugstore. Enter L'Oréal Paris True Match. Attached to its display, you'll find a plastic sheet with sample skin shades that you hold up to your face to find which hue disappears against your skin. *Voilà,* your tone!

blush powders

THE DEAL $

Sonia Kashuk Shimmering Loose Mineral Blush, in Angelica or Fairy, $8.99; www.target.com

THE ULTIMATE $$$

NARS Blush, $25; www.nars cosmetics.com

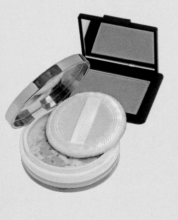

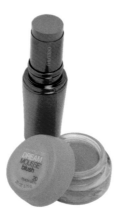

blush creams

THE DEAL $

Maybelline New York Dream Mousse Blush, $7.51; drugstores and other mass retailers

THE ULTIMATE $$$

Shiseido The Makeup Accentuating Color Stick, $30; www.sca.shiseido.com

bronzers

THE DEAL $

Physicians Formula Bronze Booster Glow-Boosting Pressed Bronzer, $14.95; drugstores and other mass retailers

THE ULTIMATE $$$

Dior Bronze Original Tan, $42; www.bloomingdales.com

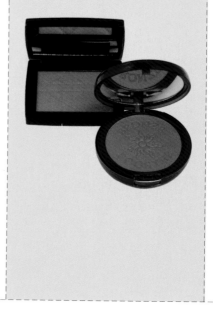

SPOTLIGHT ON HUE

The original Shimmer Brick by Bobbi Brown deserves awards for its many uses, and has inspired many imitations since it hit the shelves. I adore multiuse products, and her brick can be dabbed across eyelids, swept across cheeks, brushed on for all-over bronzing, or pinpointed on targeted spots—essentially anything you want highlighted with shimmer! When I traveled by plane, my brick broke; I put the broken slabs in a small plastic tub and used them to the very last dusting.

THE SCOOP

When to use which blush? Powder blush is ideal for all skin types and is a **save-me** for oily skin, with the highest pigment formulation. Cream blush allows some transparency to skin, but is best for those with dry skin. I avoid gel and tint blushes—you won't see them listed here—because they dry faster than I can apply them. However, once on, the "flush" they provide lasts all day long.

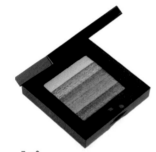

brow pencils

THE DEAL $

Physicians Formula Fineline Brow Pencil, $4.25; www.beauty.com

THE ULTIMATE $$$

Kevyn Aucoin The Precision Brow Pencil, $24; www.kevynaucoin direct.com

brow powders

THE DEAL $

e.l.f. Eyebrow Kit, $3; www.eyes lipsface.com

THE ULTIMATE $$$

Chanel Le Sourcil De Chanel Perfect Brows, $65; www.chanel.com

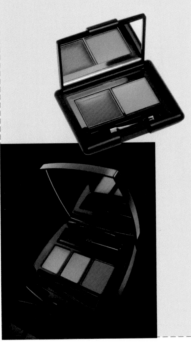

multiuse

Bobbi Brown Shimmer Brick Compact, $38; www.bobbi browncosmetics.com

other must HAVES

+ **Clear mascara used as brow gel**

+ **Self-tanner**: Clarins range of self-tanners, $32.50 to 52.50; www.us.clarins.com; or Alba Botanica Golden Tan Sunless Tanning Lotion, $9.95; www.albabotanica.com

cosmetics drawer

TRICKS OF THE TRADE

If you're on the hunt for breaking beauty news and must-know celebrity how-tos, then visit www.beautyblitz.com. Editor-in-chief and founder Polly Blitzer is a friend from our *In Style* days, and she's created a super engaging online beauty magazine that's a worthy click. Plus the site offers free, daily giveaways. Now *that's* beautiful!

APPLY THIS

For accenting your gorgeous brows, don't fret over which powder to buy. "Any matte colorstay eye shadow in an appropriate color can work as a brow powder," says Leslie Marnett. She uses Bobbi Brown Eye Shadow for both eyelids and brows ($20; www. bobbibrowncosmetics.com).

IT'S A STEAL

Hautelook, an online fashion sample sale site, also features limited flash sales on beauty products, with savings up to 75 percent off retail. Look for high-end brands like Stila, Kiehl's, and Mario Badescu Skincare. Membership is open to everyone, so log on to www. hautelook.com to save.

beautifully bronzed

A beautiful bronzer and accompanying blush with light makeup on lips and eyes, for a fresh, vibrant, sun-kissed look.

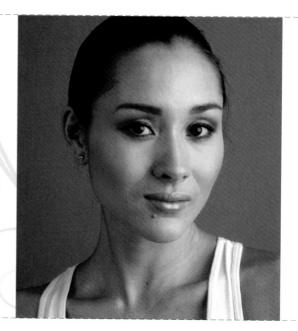

other must HAVES

+ Mally Beauty **Believable Bronzer**: $40; www.mallybeauty.com

+ Mally Beauty City Chick **Nude Lip Kit**: $25; www.mallybeauty.com

+ Mally Beauty Celebrate! **Eye Shadow**: QVC exclusive, $33; www.qvc.com

+ **Shimmer product** for highlighting face and body like Laura Mercier Loose Shimmer Powder, $34; www.lauramercier.com

+ **Pink or peach blush**

SPOTLIGHT ON HUE

Makeup artist and mother of three, Mally Roncal, who works regularly with Beyoncé, Jennifer Lopez, and Rihanna, knows how to bronze up beautifully. She advises using a matte powder bronzer without shimmer, two to three shades darker than your normal skin tone. ("Powder is easier to blend and matte is the most natural and believable looking," she says.) Bronzing is great for any skin tone. "For women of color, it can make their skin look even more alive," Roncal says.

APPLY THIS

To hide imperfections, Roncal starts with concealer applied to trouble areas, followed by foundation. Using a fluffy powder brush or blush brush with natural hair bristles, apply bronzer on the jaw line, up to just behind the ears. Continue smoothing the brush in circular motions around the perimeter of the face, hairline, temples, and hollows of the cheeks. To add depth and a more natural glow, apply a hint of blush on the apples of cheeks. Finally, to highlight, use a shimmer product on the cheek bones, across the nose, and on the brow bone.

TRICKS OF THE TRADE

For the rest of the face, Roncal suggests applying a shimmery, metallic gold or bronze to the eyelid, a couple of coats of mascara to open the eye, a beautiful pink or peach blush across the apples of the cheeks, a touch of shimmer on the cheekbones, and a light pink or nude gloss on lips. Bronze shoulders and décolletage with a shimmer product, "to accent the bones for a warm finish."

overly baked

Uneven and unnatural bronzer in a mismatched shade that isn't blended at the neck or jawline, with an un-complementary lip color.

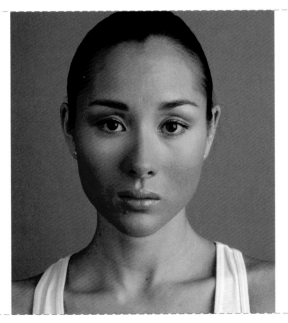

other must LOSE

— **Cream or gel bronzers** that may be difficult for the everyday woman to apply and can look patchy

— **Tanning booths** to get a fake glow

spotlight on hue

The wrong shade of bronzer can make you look dated, un-healthy, and unnatural. "The worst mistake is applying bron-zer evenly all over your face without adding blush to the apples of your cheeks," Ron-cal adds. "Forgetting that step can make the face look flat."

age alert

If you shy away from bronzer because you feel it accentuates wrinkles or crow's feet, try Ron-cal's trick: Apply a face primer underneath your foundation and then *lightly* dust on the bronzer.

apply this

"The tanorexic look is over!" exclaims Roncal. "When the bronzer exceeds two or three shades darker than your natural skin tone, you need to stop. Let's focus on a healthy glow! Our goal is to look natural." She reminds us to blend the bronzer down the jawline and throat so that face-to-neck shades are blended.

tricks of the trade

Even if you are bronzed, feel free to play up other facial fea-tures. "The rule with makeup is balance and focusing on areas you want noticed," Ron-cal says. "If the bronzer ap-plication is natural and not overpowering, then you can play up your eyes or lips and have fun with the look."

eyes

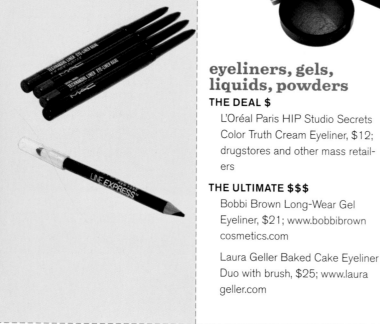

eye liners, pencils

THE DEAL $

Maybelline New York Line Express Eyeliner, $5.95; drugstores and other mass retailers

THE ULTIMATE $$$

MAC Technakohl Liner, $14.50; www.maccosmetics.com

eyeliners, gels, liquids, powders

THE DEAL $

L'Oréal Paris HIP Studio Secrets Color Truth Cream Eyeliner, $12; drugstores and other mass retailers

THE ULTIMATE $$$

Bobbi Brown Long-Wear Gel Eyeliner, $21; www.bobbibrown cosmetics.com

Laura Geller Baked Cake Eyeliner Duo with brush, $25; www.laura geller.com

eye shadows

THE DEAL $

Revlon ColorStay 12-Hour Eye Shadow Quad, $5.79; www.revlon .com for stores

THE ULTIMATE $$$

Le Métier de Beauté True Color Eye Shadow, $30; www.metier beaute.com or www.bergdorf goodman.com

Dior 5-Color Eye Shadow, from $56; www.dior.com or www.saks fifthavenue.com

THE NATURAL

Urban Decay Eyeshadow pots, $17; www.urbandecay.com

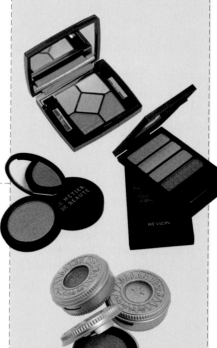

APPLY THIS

Do your watery eyes melt pencil eyeliner? Is liquid liner too defined? Consider a happy medium with a soft look that has staying power: Powder liner or shadow applied with a wet brush. Try Laura Geller Baked Cake Eyeliner Duos; www.laurageller.com.

IT'S A STEAL

Since Max Factor cosmetics stopped production and my hoarded stash was quickly used up, I've long lamented the loss of the best drugstore brand mascara on the planet: Max Factor's 2000 Calorie Mascara. Since then, I've been on the hunt for a replacement, and the verdict is L'Oréal Paris Voluminous Mascara, Original. This is a perfect example of a not-so-new product that fully delivers—up to five times fuller lashes without clumping, flaking, or anything else annoying in the lash department.

mascaras

THE DEAL $

L'Oréal Paris Voluminous Mascara, Original, $7.25; drugstores and other mass retailers

THE ULTIMATE $$$

Dior Diorshow Mascara, $24, and DiorShow Waterproof Mascara, $24; www.dior.com or www.nordstrom.com

THE NATURAL

Physicians Formula Organic wear 100% Natural Origin Mascara, $9.95; www.physiciansformula .com

Bare Escentuals Buxom Lash, $18; www.sephora.com

false lashes

THE DEAL $

Ardell Fashion Lashes, from $4.99; drugstores and other mass retailers

THE ULTIMATE $$$

Shu Uemura Natural Lashes, from $16; Sephora or www.shu uemura-usa.com

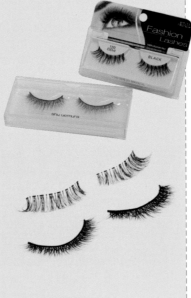

other must HAVES

+ **Eye shadow palette** that encourages experimentation: POP Beauty palettes in adorable packaging at CVS Beauty 360, from $9.99; www.cvs.com or www.popbeauty.co.uk

+ **Color mascara** that enhances eye color

+ **Shimmery shades** for highlighting and more: L'Oréal Paris HIP Studio Secrets Professional Crystal Shadow Duos, $7.99; www.loreal.com

+ **Cream eye shadow pencils**: Wet n Wild Idol Eyes Creme Eyeshadow, $1.99; drugstores and other mass retailers

THE SCOOP

A growing trend in beauty is a prestige brand developing a separate branch for the masses. For example, Hard Candy (www. hardcandy.com) hit reset and set up shop in Wal-mart. It's still a cosmetics line for the younger crowd, with eyelid tattoos, glitter gels, and Glitteratzi Body Spray. The funky packaging is alluring and they've always excelled with eye shadows, glosses, and anything involving sparkle.

style to go

Sara Strand, founder of UK-born POP Beauty, suggests using colorful, head-turning eye shadows to fulfill her company motto, "Shake up your makeup!" She traces the lash line with black or dark brown, then uses a flat or angled eyeliner brush to dot turquoise, emerald green, or a really brilliant blue eye shadow on top of it. Blend so shadows are seamless. "It makes your eyes look whiter and opens them up. People will say you look well rested!" Plus this helps balance a mature complexion that is starting to lose some hues. "Color is not about overpowering your features. It's about brightening your look, making it more modern and occasionally dramatic depending on your application."

natural looking lash boost

Fake, individual lashes that are only slightly longer than your actual lash length and appear so natural you're not sure they're even there.

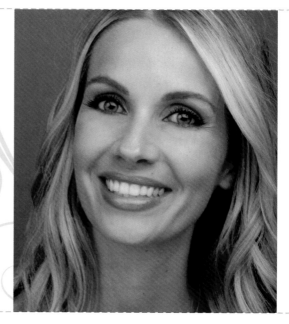

other must HAVES

+ MAC 30 Lash: **three lash lengths in one package**, $13; www.maccosmetics.com

+ Duo Clear White **Eyelash Adhesive**: $5.69; drugstores and other mass retailers

+ Ardell **Fashion Lashes** 102 Demi: dramatic for evening when trimmed to individuals, says Marnett, $3.49; drugstores and other mass retailers

+ Maybelline New York Lash Discovery **Waterproof Mascara**: has a long, lean brush and delicate application—perfect for fake lashes, $5.99; drugstores and other mass retailers

BEST BETS

Makeup artist Leslie Marnett, whose fresh-faced clients include LeAnn Rimes, Elizabeth Rohm, and Heather Graham, applies a few single lashes in the center of the lash line to help the eye pop during the day, and places a few at the outer corners of the eye for a "winged-out glamorous look" at night.

APPLY THIS

Apply eye makeup. Then curl your real lashes with an eyelash curler. Squeeze a drop of lash glue onto the back of your non-dominant hand and dip an individual lash into it to lightly cover the end. Looking downward into a mirror so your eyelid is only slightly open, grip the lash between your thumb and pinky and place it as close to the natural lash line as possible, working from the outer to inner eye corners. Repeat. Let dry for a few minutes. Apply mascara to blend the natural with the fake lashes.

THE SCOOP

Marnett's secret to a smooth application? Keeping the eye relaxed. Looking straight ahead at a mirror makes the upper eyelid taut and sensitive. But gazing downward at a mirror lets the lid relax and nearly close, thus reducing the risk of flinching.

TRICKS OF THE TRADE

Marnett uses cuticle scissors to tailor false lashes for length (opting for longer lashes toward the outer eye and shorter lashes toward the inner eye) or to take a single lash band and cut it into sections for a more controlled application. "Individual lashes are the easiest to apply with the greatest control," she says. You can use dulled tweezers to handle lashes throughout application, but only if you have steady hands!

way overdone lashes

A heavy, one-strip application of "bat wing" fake lashes topped with loads of volumizing mascara that looks more showgirl than girl next door.

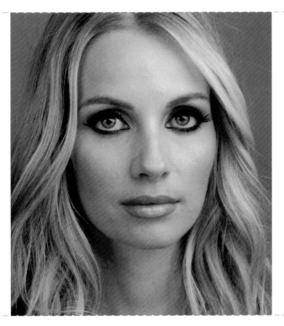

other must LOSE

— **Heavy cat-eye liquid liner** with false strip lashes

— Strong, **bold lips** with strong, **bold eyes**

— **Strip lashes so dense** that your eyelids "beat" as you blink, prepared for flight

— **Half-hanging-on strip lashes**

ditch it

"The *only* time these lashes are *ever* appropriate is when you are onstage doing toe kicks in a line with fifty other women!" exclaims Marnett. Also, the thicker and heavier the lash, the greater the chance that it will pop up. "And free-hanging renegade lashes are a major no-no!"

apply this

"Dense strip lashes make the eye look costume-ish," says Marnett. If strip lashes *are* your thing, she suggests looking for delicate, spaced-out varieties that "integrate rather than cover" your natural lashes. Use a lengthening mascara and keep other eye makeup to a minimum.

age alert

Marnett points out, "As we mature our lives often become less dramatic, and so should our makeup." Even so, false lashes are appropriate for women of all ages. Prove that you are older *and* wiser by avoiding these trying-too-hard "bat wing" lashes.

spotlight on glue

If you are heavy-handed with the white adhesive lash glue (admit it: you were that elementary schoolgirl who poured on the Elmer's!), use a black-hued glue instead. Practice will give you a better sense of how little you need: a very fine line that's as wide as the lash band.

the scoop

Should you toss lashes after one use? If you're the one donning them again, then no. Multiple wears are possible with preservation, Marnett says. Handle with care and clean off glue with a Q-tip dipped in makeup remover. Reposition the lashes in their original packaging to preserve them until the next use.

157

lips

lipsticks

THE DEAL $

Maybelline New York Color Sensational Lipcolor, $7.19; drug-stores and other mass retailers

Boots No7 Stay Perfect Lipstick or Moisture Drench Lipstick, $9.99; www.us.boots.com or www.target.com

THE ULTIMATE $$$

Giorgio Armani Sheer Lipstick, $27; www.giorgioarmanibeauty.com

Dior Addict Lipcolor, $26; www.dior.com or 866-503-9490

Chanel Rouge Coco Hydrating Crème Lip Colour, $30; www.chanel.com

THE NATURAL

Cargo PlantLove Botanical Lipstick, $20; www.cargocosmetics.com or www.beauty.com

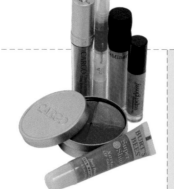

lip glosses

THE DEAL $

e.l.f. Hypershine Gloss, $1; www.eyeslipsface.com

THE ULTIMATE $$$

Philosophy the Supernatural Lip Gloss, $16.50; www.philosophy.com

Cargo Classic Lipgloss with Timestrip, $22, or Cargo Lipgloss Quad, $24; www.cargocosmetics.com or www.sephora.com

THE NATURAL

Burt's Bees Super Shiny Lip Gloss, $7; www.burtsbees.com

bareMinerals 100 % Natural Lipgloss, $15; www.bareescentuals.com

lip plumpers

THE DEAL $

Boots No7 Wild Volume Lipstick, $9.99; www.us.boots.com, Target stores or www.target.com

Estée Lauder Pure Color Gloss Sticks, $18.50; www.esteelauder.com

THE ULTIMATE $$$

DuWop Lip Venom 2nd Sin, $27; www.shop.duwop.com

THE NATURAL

Buxom Big & Healthy Lip Polish, twenty-five shades, $18; www.bareescentuals.com

Josie Maran Natural Volume Lip Gloss, $20; www.josiemaran.com

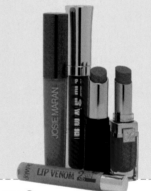

THE SCOOP

What makes lip plumpers work? Usually, ingredients that increase blood circulation in the lip. Lip-plump lovers describe this feeling as a "tingling"—just be careful the product doesn't burn. Says Leslie Marnett, "I don't believe in the stuff. It stings your lips for twenty seconds and then it's over." Her recipe for a fuller lip? Light-reflecting lip gloss, like Jordana InColor Squeeze n' Shine Super Shiny Tasty Lip Gloss, $1.99; www.jordanacosmetics.com or www.walgreens.com

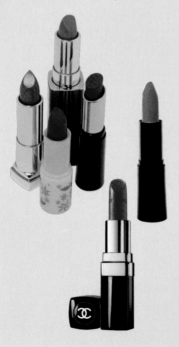

50

the number of pounds of lipstick a woman ingests over her lifetime if she applies lipstick twice a day

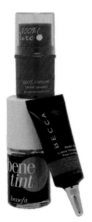

lip tints

THE DEAL $

100 Percent Pure Fruit Pigment Lip and Cheek Tint, $15; www.100percentpure.com

THE ULTIMATE $$$

Benefit Benetint, $28; www.benefitcosmetics.com

Becca Beach Tint, two-in-one crème stain for cheeks and lips, $25; www.beccacosmetics.com

lip liners

THE DEAL $

Wet n Wild Color Icon Lipliner Pencil, $.99; www.wnwbeauty.com for stores

THE ULTIMATE $$$

MAC Lip Pencil, $13; www.mac cosmetics.com

other must HAVES

+ **Clear lip liner** that goes with any shade: Mally Roncal Lip Fence, $12.50; www.mallybeauty.com

+ Go-ahead-and-eat-it **lip gloss with vitamins**: Tarte Vitamin Infused Lipgloss powered by Borba, $21; www.tartecosmetics.com

+ Silver metal **lipstick palette**, where you can stash your favorite lip colors to-go: $11.40; www.japonesque.com > palettes

APPLY THIS

Becca Cosmetics, founded by makeup artist Rebecca Morrice Williams, originally hails from Australia and has the natural look in mind. Becca Beach Tint, a versatile two-in-one for either cheeks or lips, offers a soft, luminous color that's oil-free and waterproof—a fresh alternative when your lipstick is too heavy. When I put this on, I glow like I've spent a day on the beach. And the three fruity shades—watermelon, peach, and raspberry—make me want to lick my lips because each smells like its namesake.

THE SCOOP

I have yet to find a long-wear lip color that actually lasts as long as it purports to without drying out my lips or fading. (Perhaps I like to eat, drink, and be merry too much! On TV, I certainly give my lips a workout.) The best alternative for lasting color is to apply a lip stain or tint, topped with a gloss. But you may never achieve all the pigment you crave from a full-fledged lipstick.

wear

the right red lipstick

The perfect red to complement your skin tone paired with well-balanced makeup that allows bright lips to shine.

other must HAVES

+ Barose's favorite **red lipsticks** are from MAC Cosmetics (www.maccosmetics.com), NARS (www.narscosmetics.com) and Yves Saint Laurent (www.yslbeautyus.com)

+ NARS Cosmetics **Lip Stain Gloss**, $24; www.narscosmetics.com

+ Guerlain Precious Light Rejuvenating **Illuminator**, $48; www.guerlain.com

+ Great **palette of reds** to blend and mix for your custom color: A Century in Red Lip Palette from Three Custom Color Specialists, $45; www.threecustom.com

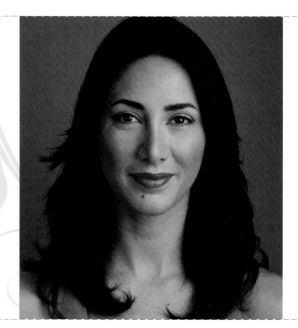

THE SCOOP

"You can rock red lips and look fresh and youthful," encourages makeup artist Nick Barose, who has painted the pouts of Anne Hathaway, Brooke Shields, and Zoe Saldana. First step: Think about texture. Too matte will age you, while super glossy smackers "can make you look like a porn star!" To strike a balance, he applies a moist, creamy lipstick with a subtle sheen that's "still somewhat sheer so you can see the natural texture of your lips peeking through."

SPOTLIGHT ON HUE

Picking the right red is crucial, but there *is* a shade of red out there for you. Barose's advice: If you are pale, go for pinky red tones; medium skin should reach for orangey reds; dark skin comes alive with berry reds. "And don't be afraid of how dark it may look in the tube," he adds.

APPLY THIS

Using a lip brush for accuracy, Barose starts from the center of lips and draws color toward the outer corners, which prevents uneven application of color and a lopsided look.

(Avoid applying from one corner to the other in one movement.) Add a few coats for more intensity. "Being precise is crucial, since any mistake shows with red lips," he warns.

TRICKS OF THE TRADE

Since Barose skips lip liner, how does he prevent color bleeding? Apply a highlighting concealer around lip lines. "Guerlain's concealer is sheer and helps brighten up the area so the color pops more." For lips that last, he dots a lip stain in a complementary hue underneath the red lipstick.

the wrong red liptstick

A red lipstick that's too bright or too dark that makes the skin look pale and unhealthy.

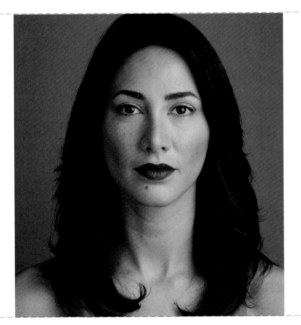

other must LOSE

- **Waxy lipstick** shades that make lips sticky
- The same **red shades you wore in your youth**

apply this

Your perfect red will fall flat if you forget to tone down the rest of your makeup. "A general rule of thumb is no severe lines: no heavy liquid eyeliner, lip liner, or contouring," says Barose. Keep your base (foundation, powder) sheer, blush a complementary pink, and eyes simple. "A face full of makeup with red lips looks tacky," Barose adds.

spotlight on hue

Opaque, heavy, and matte lips can instantly age you ten years, says Barose. Also beware of color that bleeds and feathers beyond the lip line, which makes creases and wrinkles stand out. You should wear red lips to be noticed...for the right reasons.

age alert

Red lips on an older woman can age her or make her youthful. "The key is a sheer texture with a sheen finish, and an overall balanced makeup look," says Barose. He suggests NARS Jungle Red as a starting point—"a great primary red."

the scoop

While a lip liner can define lips and keep lipstick from bleeding, the biggest mistake is lining lips with a matching red lip pencil. If you're lining your lips, try a nude shade that is "softer, more natural," says Barose. If you have a decent natural lip shade, avoid lip liner at all costs.

ditch it

Never match your nails to red lipstick—that's old fashioned, says Barose. Go for nail colors like nudes and sheer pinks or dark wines and berries.

tools

eyelash curlers

THE DEAL $

e.l.f. Mechanical Eyelash Curler, $1; www.eyeslipsface.com

Revlon Professional Eyelash Curler, $3.99; www.revlon.com

THE ULTIMATE $$$

Shu Uemura Eyelash Curler, $19; www.shuuemura-usa.com

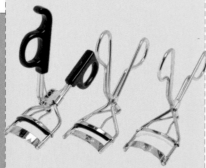

tweezers

THE DEAL $

Revlon Expert Tweezer Square Tip, $6.40; drugstores and other mass retailers

THE ULTIMATE $$$

Tweezerman Slant Tweezer, nine colors, $20; www.tweezerman.com

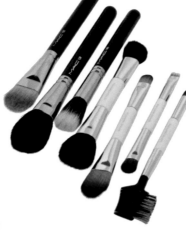

makeup brushes

THE DEAL $

Sonia Kashuk, assorted brushes, from $4.99; www.target.com

THE ULTIMATE $$$

MAC, assorted brushes, from $11; www.maccosmetics.com

brow kit

Anastasia Beverly Hills Brow Tool Kit, $45; www.anastasia.net.

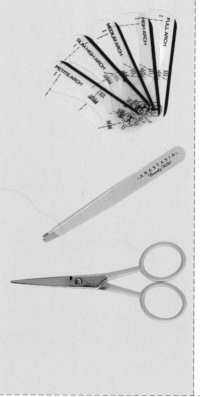

BEST BETS

Confession: I didn't start tweezing my eyebrows until I started working in magazines. It's not that I didn't know better; I simply liked my bushy brows as a natural alternative. But after a few tweezes—for a story—I reveled in how a tailored brow makes your eyes pop and opens the entire look of your face. If you are a brow newbie like I once was and want to DIY, try a brow kit by celebrity aesthetician Anastasia to get your uncharted plucking on course.

makeup sponges

THE DEAL $

Essence of Beauty Rounds or Wedges, $3.49; www.cvs.com

THE ULTIMATE $$$

BeautyBlender sponge, $19.95; www.amazon.com or www.beauty-blender.net for information

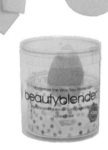

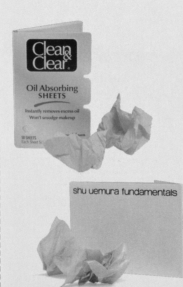

matte blotting papers

THE DEAL $

Clean & Clear Oil-Absorbing Sheets, $5.49; drugstores and other mass retailers

THE ULTIMATE $$$

Shu Uemura Face Paper, $12; www.shuuemura-usa.com

other must HAVES

+ Brush Off **brush cleaner**, $9; www.brushoff.com

+ **Mild shampoo** and water to hand-wash your makeup brushes

+ Face **Waterproof Eye Makeup Remover**, $10; www.sephora.com

the Scoop

What's all the fuss about mineral makeup? Formulated from natural, pure, micronized minerals, it tends to have no oils, dyes, preservatives, fillers, binders, silicones, chemicals, or wax…ingredients known to be skin irritants, which is why it's great for sensitive skin types. Mineral makeup not only hides your flaws but also allows your skin to breathe. It's one of the hottest trends in makeup!

APPLY THIS

Since you use makeup brushes every day, it's important to clean them. The no-fuss method: Wash them with warm water and a mild detergent such as shampoo and allow to air dry. Or use a specially formulated makeup brush cleanser. Pros say to wash every three months. I say, if you use your brushes as furiously and frequently as I do, cleanse at least once a month while watching the news or a favorite show.

TRICKS OF THE TRADE

I was exposed to oil-blotting papers long before they hit the United States, as they're a Japanese beauty ritual. Originally used to absorb oil and sweat atop the traditional white cake makeup of dancers, theater actors, or geisha, today's blotters, like Shu Uemura's, serve the same purpose: to lift off the oil while leaving makeup intact.

wear

natural

The five-minute miracle make-under—a beautiful blend of natural-looking makeup to perfectly enhance your favorite facial features and give you an overall glow.

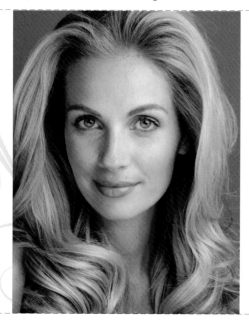

other must HAVES

+ **Well-groomed brows**—thin brows age you
+ **Cream blush** that doubles as a lip stain—save time and money
+ For the dexterous, **mascara that doubles as eyeliner**
+ **Bronzer** instead of an overly pink blush

APPLY THIS

Makeup artist Leslie Marnett knows that a little makeup can go a long way for a fresh, clean look. To a moisturized face, apply concealer under the eyes and around the nose and chin. Dust powder foundation over your entire face. Sweep blush from the apples of the cheeks out toward the ears. Trace eyeliner along the line of your top lid from the inner to the outer corners. From the outer corners, lightly work the eyeliner three-quarters of the way along your bottom lashes. Apply two coats of mascara to the top lashes and one coat to the bottom (eyeliner and mascara should be black or brown for this look). Finish with two swipes of tinted lip balm.

TRICKS OF THE TRADE

Sometimes being hands-on with makeup means putting brushes aside. With this look, Marnett suggests using your ring finger to both apply concealer and blend eyeliner so the edges are soft.

THE SCOOP

To give an instant lift, Marnett applies light-reflecting concealer to the inner corners of the eyes and dabs a lip gloss that reflects light in the center of lips to make pouts look plump and youthful. Another eye-opening trick: Wear eyeliner in a shade that closely matches the ring around your iris.

AGE ALERT

This look works for *most* ages. "As we age, our natural coloring tends to fall a little flat," warns Marnett. "So if you need a little more oomph, add a rosy blush or take your lip a touch brighter."

A makeup-free face, revealing oily, dry, pasty, or chalky skin, highlighting problem areas, dark circles, or sunken eyes.

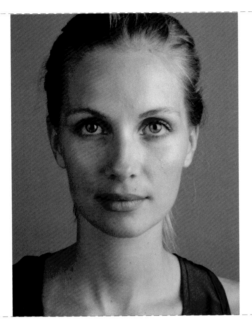

other must LOSE

— **Oily skin,** uncared-for looks

— Not playing up your facial assets

— **Discolorations, redness, ruddiness**

apply this

Until we locate the fountain of youth, we should embrace make-up for what it can hide—from under-eye circles to stressed skin. Says Marnett, "Makeup can make us look put together, even on days when we can barely put together a sentence!"

tricks of the trade

Lack of time is no excuse for not wearing makeup. Want to look more awake after a restless night? Concealer and mascara is all you need, Marnett shares. Have an interview? Groomed brows, even skin tone, and healthy cheek color reveal a confident, composed woman. "Whether you want to conceal or enhance, use makeup to do so in a matter of minutes."

ditch it

During the day, fatigue and oil start to show on your face. "Remember, skin is an organ," Marnett reminds. "It needs to be fed (skincare) and protected (cosmetics) just like anything else on your body." If zero or minimal makeup is your goal, then your daily skin routine *must* take priority, so at the very least, your skin's in peak condition.

age alert

A little makeup *can* be your ticket to a youthful appearance. "Our skin tells the story of our lives, which showcases stress, wrinkles, and sun spots obtained from life," Marnett says. Solutions: illuminating concealers and foundations, fresh cheek colors, and juicy lip textures. "Most importantly, the confidence we exude by putting our best face forward is beauty no one can re-create."

replacing makeup

Though we don't want to admit it, our newly revamped cosmetics drawer is now expiring as we speak. *What*? Makeup, like food, has expiration dates. *Who in the heck follows these dates*? you ask. Everybody should. Because bacteria build up in our everyday products and can lead, in the worst case, to rashes and infections.

The good news is right under your nose: Many products have expiration dates stamped right on them. Look on the packaging for a little tub icon that has a number on it like 6M, 12M, 24M, 36M (see examples below). That tells you how many months the product should last from the time you open it.

For those products without the handy expiration labeling, the chart on the next page lists general guidelines. Keep in mind that all-natural products have far fewer preservatives and will expire even sooner. Consult the store or manufacturer to find out your product's expiration timeframe.

Here's a tip: Place a small sticker on the product and write the month and year (such as 4/2011) you open it. Better yet, calculate the date it *expires* and write that down. And if anything has a strange odor or is starting to separate, crackle, or clump, *just toss it!*

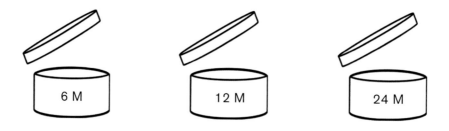

6 M   12 M   24 M

how long should you keep it?

makeup

CONCEALER	1 year
FOUNDATION	1–1½ years
FACIAL POWDER	2 years
BLUSH, POWDER	2 years
BLUSH, CREAM	1 year
BRONZER	2 years
PENCIL EYELINER	2 years
LIQUID EYELINER	3 months
EYE SHADOW, POWDER	2 years
EYE SHADOW, CREAM	1 year
MASCARA	3 months
BROW LINER OR POWDER	2 years
LIPSTICK	2 years
LIP GLOSS	1½–2 years
LIP LINER	up to 3 years, if pencil
MAKEUP BRUSHES	wash every 3 months with a brush cleanser
NAIL POLISH	2 years

skincare products

CLEANSER	1 year
MIST	1 year
MOISTURIZERS	1 year
EYE CREAM	1 year
SUNSCREEN	1 year
MAKEUP PRIMER	6 months–1 year
LIP BALM	1 year
EXFOLIATORS	6-9 months
ANTI-AGING MASQUES & TREATMENTS	6 months–1 year

cosmetics drawer

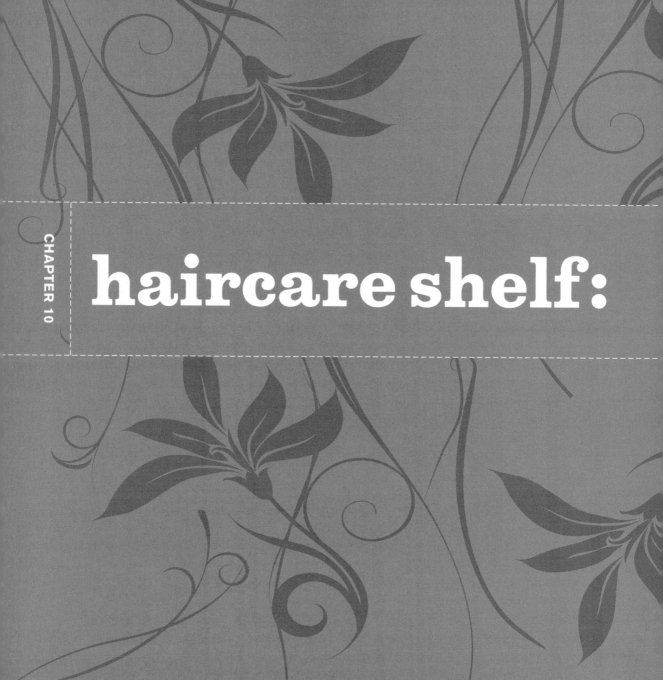

haircare shelf:

cleansing & conditioning, styling products, hair tools

cleansing & conditioning

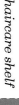

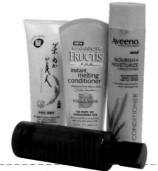

shampoos

THE DEAL $

Pantene Pro-V Classic Shampoo, $3.99; drugstores and other mass retailers

THE LITTLE LUXURY $$

Joico Daily Care Balancing Shampoo for Normal Hair, $10.99; drugstores and other mass retailers

THE ULTIMATE $$$

Kérastase Bain Satin 1, $34; www.kerastase-usa.com

conditioners

THE DEAL $

Aveeno + Nourish Conditioner (moisturize, revitalize, or volumize formulas), $6.99; drugstores and other mass retailers

Garnier Fructis Instant Melting Conditioner, $4.29; drugstores and other mass retailers

THE LITTLE LUXURY $$

Komenuka Bijin Moisturizing Hair Treatment, $33; www.komenuka-bijin.com or 877-737-4247

THE ULTIMATE $$$

Shu Uemura Full Shimmer Illuminating Conditioner, $55; www.shuuemuraartofhair-usa.com

ever wonder how old your hair is?

The average person's hair grows about a half-inch per month. And, as your hair grows longer, it ages. This means that a section ten inches down from the root is almost two years old.

THE SCOOP

Do we *need* a weekly deep hair treatment? "Basically, what you are really doing is spending more money to get the same thing as your regular conditioner," says Paula Begoun, the Cosmetics Cop. "But the longer you keep a conditioner on, the better coverage you get in and around the cuticle—not penetration into the actual hair, but better coverage in and around the outer layer of the hair—and that's nice."

TRICKS OF THE TRADE

Celebrity hairstylist Kevin Mancuso actually recommends a deep conditioning treatment every *two weeks* to help control damage caused by styling. "Women with fine hair can apply the treatment to the hair tips if they are scared that a heavy or deep conditioner will weigh hair down," he says.

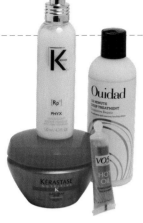

deep treatments

THE DEAL $

Alberto V05 Hot Oil Moisturizing Treatment, a weekly intense conditioning treatment, $3.99 for two; www.amazon.com

THE LITTLE LUXURY $$

Ouidad Deep Treatment, $25; www.ouidad.com

THE ULTIMATE $$$

Kérastase Masque Oléo Relax Slim, $60; www.kerastase-usa.com

Kronos Phyx Overnight Hair Masque, $105; www.kronos hair.com

THE BIG BANG THEORY!

STRAIGHT HAIR

The best candidate for bangs, but still requires trimming and styling. A disheveled bang can throw off your whole look.

CURLY HAIR

Consider a shorter frame and no full-on bangs. If you plan to wear your bangs straight, you need to straighten your hair…every day.

SMALL FOREHEAD

Skip the bang. You need the distance between your hairline and eyebrow to be open and uninterrupted

"SUBURBAN BANG"

This is a thin bang that disconnects entirely from the rest of the haircut and instantly ages women. "It is a calling card that says, 'I live in the suburbs and I have lines on my forehead that I want to hide,'" says Arturo. Grow out the corners and connect them to the rest of the frame of the cut, so hair flows all together as one soft, flowing unit.

---

other must HAVES

+ **Dry shampoo**, a **save-me** for between washings: Oscar Blandi Pronto Dry Shampoo Spray, $11; www.sephora.com

+ Shampoo/conditioner that **combats dandruff**

+ Weekly **clarifying shampoo:** Charles Worthington Results Well Balanced Shampoo, $6, or Neutrogena Anti-Residue Shampoo, $5.99; drugstores and other mass retailers

---

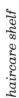

BEST BETS

Komenuka Bijin is my under-the-radar Asian cleansing secret. In Japan, it is sold at drugstores, and here you can get it online. The Moisturizing Hair Shampoo is so luxurious your hair feels softer just by massaging it in. After rinsing the shampoo out, the conditioner is like icing on the cake, and makes my dry tresses bouncy and silky soft.

APPLY THIS

There's more you can do to soften hair than simply applying conditioner. Mancuso suggests using a natural bristle brush on dry hair to promote and distribute the scalp's natural oils, which begs the question, *how often should you wash that beneficial oil out*? "The answer depends on your personal hair texture and what ultimately works for you for best results," he says. Generally, women with finer hair should wash more frequently because excess oil can weigh down the hair. Women with thicker hair can wash less frequently since their hair tends to be drier to begin with.

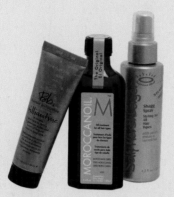

normal to dry

THE DEAL $
Sally Hershberger Supreme Head Shag Spray, $12.50; drugstores and other mass retailers

THE LITTLE LUXURY $$
Bumble and Bumble Brilliantine, $20; www.bumbleandbumble.com

THE ULTIMATE $$$
The Original MoroccanOil Treatment, $39; www.moroccanoil.com or fine salons

straight

THE DEAL $
Paul Mitchell Super Skinny Serum, $16.95; www.paulmitchell.com or Paul Mitchell salons

THE LITTLE LUXURY $$
Fekkai Coiff Controle Ironless Straightening Balm, $25; www.fekkai.com

THE ULTIMATE $$$
Phyto Phytovolume Actif Volumizer Spray, $28; www.phyto-usa.com

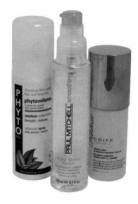

10
the number of inches of hair needed to donate to Locks of Love, an organization that provides hairpieces for children suffering from long-term medical hair loss.

TRICKS OF THE TRADE
During its debut this product generated so much buzz that it sold out worldwide! Shu Uemura Art of Hair Essence Absolue hair oil ($48, www.shuuemuraartofhair-usa.com) is an elixir for dry hair that you can use for a multitude of purposes—from styling blowouts to controlling flyaways to securing weightless curls. Hey, if it's good enough for Jennifer Aniston's tresses…

BEST BETS
Ever wonder how curly your curls are? A fascinating function of Mizani's site (www.mizani-usa.com) is its Natural Curl Key. Here, global hair types have been scientifically sorted into eight categories, from straight to zigzag coiled. Find your type, get the low-down on its properties, and discover corresponding Mizani products to treat your locks. Mizani, which was started in 1991, initially targeted African-American consumers and now designs products for all hair types under L'Oréal USA.

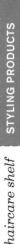

curly

THE DEAL $

John Frieda Collection Frizz-Ease Serum Original Formula, $9.99; drugstores and other mass retailers

THE LITTLE LUXURY $$

Nexxus Salon Hair Care Lavish Body, $10.55; drugstores and other mass retailers

Nexxus Salon Hair Care Thermal Volume, $10.55; drugstores and other mass retailers

THE ULTIMATE $$$

Ouidad Climate Control Heat and Humidity Gel, $22; www.ouidad.com

MoroccanOil Intense Curl Cream, $30; www.moroccanoil.com or fine salons

style to go

"Adding a beautiful hair accessory to a bun is one of the easiest ways to update the look," says Kevin Mancuso. He adds a bejeweled hair comb or a fresh flower for an instant polished finish. "Placing the accessory on the top or side of the bun tends to be more playful and casual, while a lower placement produces a more elegant look."

other must HAVES

+ Amazing **hairspray**: Tigi Bed Head Hard Head Hard Hold Hairspray, $15; www.tigihaircare.com for information

+ A **diffuser** add-on for your hair dryer to enhance curly hair: Hot Sock Ultralight Diffuser, $4.95; www.folica.com

THE SCOOP

Perhaps you've heard of Hercut, a haircare line that addresses hair styles rather than hair types. It's an interesting approach, particularly when many stylists say that understanding hair texture is the most important aspect of purchasing maintenance and styling products. Categorized by classic cuts (The Bob, The Blunt, The Shag, The Long Layers, and The Pixie), Hercut offers styling products formulated to bring out the best in each cut. Shampoos and conditioners are also available (www.hercut.com or www.sephora.com).

hair tools

hair dryers

THE DEAL $

BaByliss Pro Ceramix Extreme Hair Dryer, $45; www.folica.com or www.babylisspro.co.uk for information

THE LITTLE LUXURY $$

The Original Super Solano Hair Dryer, $145; www.solanopower.com

THE ULTIMATE $$$

T3 Bespoke Labs Featherweight Professional Hair Dryer, $200; www.t3micro.com

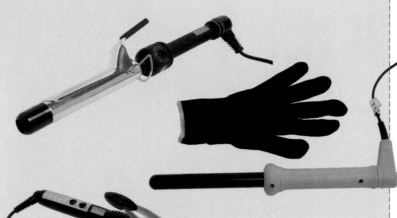

curling irons

THE DEAL $

Infiniti by Conair Infiniti Curling Irons, from $26.99; www.conair.com

THE LITTLE LUXURY $$

Hot Tools Professional Jumbo 1-inch Curling Iron by Folica, $34; www.folica.com

THE ULTIMATE $$$

Enzo Milano 19-mm Curling Iron (¾-inch curl), $119; www.shop enzomilano.com

BEST BETS

With more than a decade on the web, Folica (www.folica.com) is a trusted, non-hair-raising site for shopping for hair products, styling tools, and more. The buyer guides are ranked according to customer reviews, and the top ten lists can help out those who are clueless.

IT'S A STEAL

Fashion flash sale sites have skyrocketed in popularity, and now beauty-exclusive sites are getting in on the action. Beauty Ticket (www.beautyticket.com) sells premium beauty brands like Prada and Yves Saint Laurent for up to 85 percent off. No membership required.

TRICKS OF THE TRADE

Most of us think flat irons are just for straightening hair. Wrong! Versatile models, like the popular, designer-beloved ghd IV styler, sport rounded barrels that can actually create curls and twists. Most high-end irons have a certain number of bells and whistles, and this one does as well:

flat irons

THE DEAL $

Infiniti by Conair You Style Multi-functional Styling Iron, $44.99; www.conair.com or mass retailers

THE LITTLE LUXURY $$

Chi USA Original Ceramic HS Flatiron, $159.97; www.chiretail.com

THE ULTIMATE $$$

ghd IV Styler—ceramic 1-inch styling iron, $240; www.ghdhair.com/us

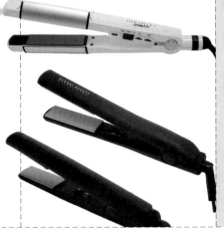

hairbrushes

THE DEAL $

Spornette, from $6.75; www.spornette.com

THE LITTLE LUXURY $$

Denman, from $8.99; www.denmanbrush.com

THE ULTIMATE $$$

Mason Pearson, from $50; www.neimannmarcus.com or www.masonpearson.com for information

other must HAVES

+ To **stop hair breakage and revive dry and damaged hair**, use twice a month: Nexxus Emergencée Strengthening Polymeric Reconstructor, $19.99; drugstores and other mass retailers

+ To **clean hair on the go**: Ted Gibson Hair Sheet, $14.99; www.tedgibsonsalon.com

automatic shut-off, evenly heated ceramic plates that infuse moisture to the hair shaft, and safe but intense heat that flattens or curls hair in seconds.

BEST BETS

If you like reading reviews from fellow beauty lovers, www.totalbeauty.com is your ultimate web site. It tallies unbiased reviews by real women and provides a forum for discussing thousands of products: the good, the bad, the must-gets, and the avoids! You save money by learning what to steer clear of.

TRICKS OF THE TRADE

Your tools are the most important part of getting a perfect end result and the same applies to home blowouts," says celebrity stylist Arturo of Arturo New York. His professional **save-me** recommendations for your beauty box are Grip Clips by Lucky, a professional grade blow dryer, and hair brushes by Marilyn Brushes.

from the mouths of mavens: **PAULA BEGOUN**

If you ever want the low-down on beauty, skin, and hair products, Paula Begoun, consumer advocate, is the person to call. Her web site, www.beautypedia.com, features tens of thousands of product reviews, all written with her signature candor and supporting studies that back up her claims. You will marvel at her knowledge and at what you didn't know about haircare.

THE DIRTY ON HAIR

How often should we be washing our hair?

For the majority of people, as infrequently as possible. The very acts of washing, brushing, and styling are damaging to hair. Nothing you do can prevent this.

Why does hair get heavy, oily, and limp?

If you are using a volumizing, moisturizing, or conditioning shampoo or a shampoo for dry or damaged hair, they almost always contain conditioning or hairspray-like ingredients that can build up on hair. You want to wash them out completely every three to four shampoos with a clarifying shampoo.

Once and for all, it is time to debunk the myth that hair adapts to shampoo.

If you find your hair starting to get limp after the use of an otherwise effective shampoo that you like, use a clarifying shampoo once a week to remove any excess buildup. With your next wash, your hair will bounce back and be ready for your favorite shampoo.

You have very specific tips about how to use conditioner.

Apply conditioner about an inch to an inch and a half from the root of the hair. Unless you have a dry scalp, using conditioner on the root of your hair—which is new hair and doesn't need it—can weigh hair down. You can help your hair feel healthy, depending on the products you use and how you use them. So put conditioner on your oldest, least healthy part of your hair—the ends.

What conditions lead to dry scalp?

Dry scalp occurs when your scalp doesn't produce much oil or you are over-drying your hair, swimming every day, or over-exposing your hair to the sun. People feel the need to wash their hair every day, or wash twice through, or let their blow dryer get too close to their scalp. Preventing dry scalp is more about what *not* to do rather than what to do.

What's an effective treatment for dry scalp?

If you know you'll wash your hair in the morning, take your hair conditioner and massage it into the dry areas of the scalp at night as a treatment while you sleep.

Let's talk about trends in products and product ingredients. What do we make of the new products that claim to be sulfate-free?

There is nothing about sulfates that is a problem. There is only one sulfate that you need be wary of if it appears in a product's list of ingredients: sodium lauryl sulfate. While it is an extremely effective cleanser for the hair, it also is a strong irritant and can therefore irritate and dry out the scalp. Cocamidopropyl betaine, often found in baby shampoos, is increasingly being used in adult shampoos; it is an effective yet gentle and mild cleanser.

Any benefit to vitamins in shampoos?

A shampoo can be filled with vitamins but that won't improve your hair. Hair is dead so it can't be nourished. Silicones will make it shiny, proteins might fill damaged cuticles, but there is no such thing as vitamins that "nourish" or "feed" your hair. Even if vitamins did benefit hair in some way, they would be rinsed down the drain before they had a chance to work.

On that note, many shampoos claim to have UV filters and sun protection. Are there products you recommend for hair protection when it comes to sun exposure?

A hat! That's why there are no haircare products with an SPF rating. Sunscreen can't stand up against rinsing and washing and styling your hair with heat. Those ingredients break down.

We love products that smell good. Are fragranced essential oil products good for hair?

Essential oils smell wonderful, but in hair products they are plain old irritants. In fact, fragrance can be the number one irritant, making the scalp itchy, red, and inflamed. What I ask people to consider is this: If you decide to wear a fragrance or cologne, put that same fragrance on your hair so you don't have different scents competing with one other.

Are shampoos for color-treated hair a myth?

These shampoos don't lock in color to the hair shaft any better than a normal shampoo. They contain no ingredients that differ from other shampoos. Once in a while they may contain synthetic dyes, but these can't remain on hair or penetrate the hair shaft.

Are different hair-designated types of shampoos pointless?

Don't buy a shampoo that says for "curly," "straight," or "frizzy" hair. Why? You wash the shampoo out; how effective can that be? Treating hair types really happens with the styling product. That's where you buy the mousse to enhance the curl, the balm to help straighten, and the spray to reduce static or frizz.

So styling products are the best way to deal with curly, dry, straight, thick and coarse, fine and thin hair?

Yes. You will find that, for the most part, the styling product will do what it advertises. It is true, however (and this is a very big however), that results mostly depend on your hairstyling technique. In other words, if you use a product that says it is going to curl your hair, it sure isn't going to curl your hair without a curling iron or a really good round brush. If it is going to straighten your hair, we all know that without a really good flat iron you aren't getting Jennifer Aniston hair. Even Jennifer Aniston hair isn't getting Jennifer Aniston hair!

So hair is really far more about styling technique, and the styling products are an adjunct.

Speaking of technique, earlier you mentioned blow drying too close to the scalp. Is there a right distance?

It isn't really about how close but about how quickly you move the heat through your hair. The average blow dryer and flat iron heat up to almost 400 degrees because this is the temperature level that changes, alters, and controls the shape of hair. The trick is never to linger over the hair. When you look at a great hair stylist at work, you never see him or her holding the heat in one place for very long.

Do you have a parting thought about price?

Let me say this unequivocally and without hesitation: There is no need to pay over $10 for a generous size of hair product. More expensive brands often have the exact same formulations as drugstore brands. The few plant extracts or vitamins that get thrown in are rinsed down the drain and are a waste of money, so you are paying for the marketing.

haircare shelf

wear

LAYERS
Arturo

haircare shelf

FACE-FLATTERING LAYERS

face-flattering layers

Delicious layers that work with hair density, weight, and volume and suit face shape, cheekbones, and neck length.

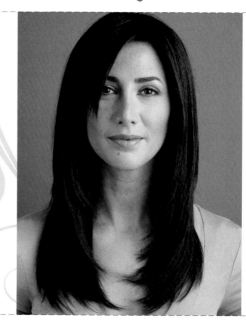

other must HAVES

+ Super short do with **fun pixie layers**
+ **Hairspray that doesn't flake**: L'Oréal Elnett Satin Hairspray Extra Strong Hold, $14.99; drugstores and other mass retailers
+ Darker hair color and layers creates the appearance of **more body for thinning hair**

THE SCOOP

With layers, the fringe benefits are huge. "Layers take the bulk out of thick, mushrooming hair and add body to thin and medium hair," says celebrity hair stylist Arturo of Arturo New York, who has styled Shakira, Julia Roberts, and Arianna Huffington. "They frame the face, adding softness, movement, and sexiness." Aim for an even look with no gaps between layers, so the entire frame of the hair flows together from back to front.

AGE ALERT

Layers are for everyone, says Arturo. "I don't believe in the unwritten rule that states women of a certain age should wear their hair short. Every face shape can benefit from layering."

APPLY THIS

Bring photos of layers you love to your stylist. Discuss and be realistic about your hair type and what you can achieve. "Start by getting long layers so you can understand the styling it takes to maintain them," advises Arturo. "Then you can always take your layers a little shorter until you find the perfect length that works for you."

ever wonder who your hair pinup gal should be?

While layering techniques abound, the head to turn to for the best layers in recent years is Heidi Klum. "Sometimes she wears her frame longer, sometimes a little shorter, giving the effect of a long bang," says Arturo. Either way, it's perfection.

toss

the bad straight cut

A messy-edged straight cut that is utterly disheveled and not maintained.

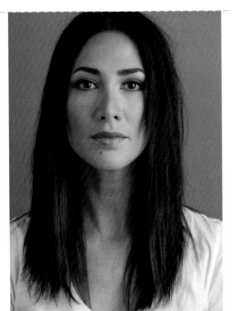

other must LOSE

- **Volumizing hair products**—look for products that straighten and add shine instead
- Stark, **angular cut on an angular face**
- **Straight cut for super thick hair**

ditch it

Don't play a numbers game with layers. "I love it when women say they want three layers in back!" laughs Arturo. "Bad layering is when the hair looks disconnected and falls in random chunks around the head, like someone took out a hedge mower and hacked away."

tricks of the trade

A blunt cut has to be cut perfectly straight to make a statement. Hair must be in top-notch condition, as in super shiny and blown out to dead straight perfection, to really steal the show. It's a high-maintenance look, says Arturo, who points to Katie Holmes, circa 2010, as the primo example with her sleek, perfectly groomed, strong, symmetrical line. "When it's done right," he adds, "it is a runway show for healthy hair."

best bets

A blunt, straight cut can look exceptional and works best for women with very fine, limp hair. Most commonly, women go for a bob, which helps hair look thicker. Another option is a 1960s retro chic straight cut, parted down the middle. If you have naturally straight hair, consider this cut.

ultimate blowout

A pristine, beautiful blowout that makes hair look shiny, healthy, and gorgeous.

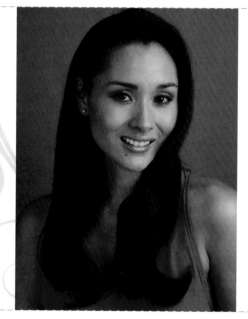

other must HAVES

+ For **added body**: Kérastase Spray Volumactive, $36; www.kerastase-usa.com

+ **Anti-frizz on medium to thick hair**: Kérastase Sérum Oléo-Relax, $36

+ For **thick, unruly hair**: Kérastase Elixir Oléo-Relax, $36

+ To **create volume for thinning hair**: Lotion Densitive GL by Kérastase, $41

+ For oily hair, use a **dry shampoo** like Naturia by Rene Furterer ($12; www.sephora.com) to help the blowout last longer

APPLY THIS

Arturo, the creator of iBlow—a step-by-step at-home blow-dry technique—shares his expert tips for the perfect blowout. Towel-dry hair by squeezing, not excessive rubbing, with a towel. Apply a protective styling product according to your hair type (see Best Bets). Section the hair into bundles no thicker than two inches, no wider than four inches, and clip up each section. Start at the back of the head and work through the sides toward the top of head. One section at a time, place your brush securely at the underside of the roots, grip the hair with the bristles, and start blowing hair down. As you travel the length of the hair, point the air from the dryer in the same direction as the brush. Repeat this motion a couple times until that section of hair is totally smooth and dry. Move to the next section. Repeat. When you're at the crown of the head, blow the air straight up with the hair blowing back, away from your face. Sparingly apply a finishing styling product to secure the shape and control flyaways.

BEST BETS

Arturo, a distributor for Kérastase, recommends the following Kérastase pre-blowout styling products applied to towel-dried tresses: For thin hair, Lotion Densitive GL, and for medium hair, Spray Volumactive, sprayed onto the roots and lightly on the midshaft before blow-drying every section; for thick hair, Sérum Oléo-Relax, and for thick/unruly hair, Elixir Oléo-Relax, worked from the hair ends upward toward the roots, then combed through for even distribution before starting your blowout.

THE SCOOP

For adding body, blow your roots in the opposite direction from how you want hair to fall, says Arturo. Or, after finishing each section of blow-dried hair, wrap the hair ends around the brush, blast with heat for a few seconds, and then release for added bounce.

natural air dry

Uncontrollable bedhead hair that is messy and tangled—a bird's nest.

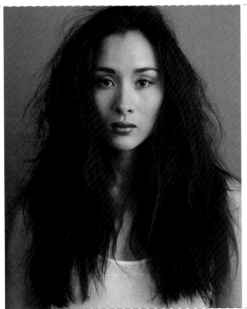

other must LOSE

- **Unbrushed hair** (unless it's super curly)
- Hair with **excessive tangles** that bunch up to create knots
- **Overly hairsprayed hair** to the point of helmet head

ditch it

While air drying is the most healthy alternative for hair, when left untouched it can be unruly. Arturo insists, "You need to start by getting a great cut that works with your hair type. Next, invest in some styling products that will tame and condition your hair." He warns that hair without product rarely works, so don't do it.

the scoop

Walking around with unblown hair is a drippy downer. "If you're walking around with your hair wet, it's only because you have the right products in your hair and you know what you are doing to achieve the overall look when it actually dries. Otherwise, it's a huge no-no," Arturo says.

apply this

There is such a thing as styling hair to look "naturally dried" like Kate Moss' locks, and Arturo insists it is simple to achieve. First add volumizing mousse to your already dried hair. Take a 1½-inch curling iron and unscrew the handle; all you need is the pole (or simply keep the handle pressed open while you style). Now, wrap sections of hair around the iron, starting about three inches away from the root and going away from the face. Hold for a few seconds, then pull the hair down to stretch it out. Repeat with random sections until all the hair on your head is wavy. Then rub some shine product in your hands, grab hair sections, and squeeze and tousle away, "until you look like you belong in a Victoria's Secret campaign."

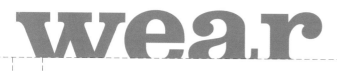

wear

natural beach waves

Hair in tousled, piecy waves that look like you've spent the day at the shore.

other must HAVES

+ To prep hair for styling and offer protection from hot styling tools: Sally Hershberger Supreme Head **Style Primers for Wavy Hair,** $12.50; www.sallyhershberger.com

+ **Mineral spray** for the wind-blown hair look: Sally Hershberger Salon Mineral Spray Styler, $24; www.hsn.com

+ For a **fresh, tousled beachy look and smell**: Bumble and Bumble Surf Spray, $25.99; drugstores and other mass retailers

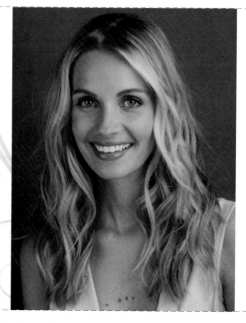

THE SCOOP

"When I think of natural beachy hair, I think of Gisele Bundchen, she rocks it!" says celebrity hairstylist Sally Hershberger, who has cut the locks of Julia Roberts, Renée Zellweger, and Tom Cruise. Hershberger loves this look with any hair length and face shape. "Because of its natural movement, you can divert attention away from imperfections, like eyes set close together or a low or short jaw. It is very versatile."

APPLY THIS

Apply a mousse to damp hair and comb through the hair to distribute evenly throughout. With a hairdryer, rough dry the hair with your fingers until it's 90 percent dry. Blow the last 10 percent dry with a round brush to create body and shine. Wrap sections of hair around a 1½- or 2-inch curling iron to create a loose wave. Curl both small and big sections of hair for a more natural flow to the overall look. "Remember to keep the curls balanced on both sides of the face; the rest of the head can be random curl formations," says Hershberger. Spritz a wave-enhancing spray and a mineral spray to get that slightly unkempt, sea-salty look.

TRICKS OF THE TRADE

Use a shampoo and conditioner that enhance texture to achieve this look," Hershberger says. Also, don't hold the hair on the iron for a long time or the curls will be too tight.

BEST BETS

Super straight hair can wear waves, too. Following the steps in Apply This, Hershberger also spritzes thermal setting spray to wet straight hair before blow-drying to protect it from the heat of styling tools and to help the curl last longer.

wear

Sexy, voluminous curls that go all the way around the head.

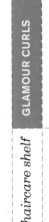

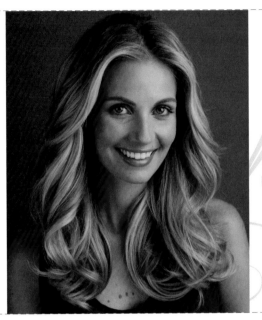

other must HAVES

+ Mason Pearson **wide-tooth rake comb**, $28; www.bergdorfgoodman.com

+ **Leave-in thermal protective** product that softens hair: Chi Silk Infusion, $22.99; www.amazon.com

+ **Hot rollers**: BaByliss Pro Ceramic 20 Roller Set, $54.95; www.folica.com

APPLY THIS

Starting at the crown of the head and working toward the ends, apply volumizing mousse and a curl-enhancing style product to wet hair, scrunching with your hands rather than combing it through. Make a deep side part into the hair and blow dry, preserving the part and using your fingers to scrunch the hair upward toward the scalp. For defined curls, use a standard, spring-loaded-handle curling iron (a smaller barrel, ½ to 1 inch, for tight curls; a larger barrel, 1½ to 2 inches, for looser curls) to shape curls around the face. For enhanced hold, after curling a section of hair with the curling iron, coil each curl into a small circle and clip or pin in place. Once your hair is cooled and set, remove the clips. Hershberger likes to brush out the curls using a wide-tooth comb or her fingers to connect the curls and enhance body and flow.

TRICKS OF THE TRADE

Another way to get glamour curls is by using hot rollers on dry hair. First, apply a thermal protective spray. Using the biggest rollers in the set, begin rolling at the top of the head. Wrap a two- to three-inch section of hair and tuck the ends around the roller, rolling back away from your forehead. Look for sets with large clips that clamp over the entire roller for a secure hold. Work back, curling the top sections of hair so the rollers are lined up in a row atop the crown. Following the same technique, roll the hair on the sides of the head and the bottom near the nape of the neck until the entire head is completely rolled (rollers should always lie in vertical rows). Mist with hairspray. Allow to cool, then remove the rollers and comb your fingers through the curls to blend.

wear

good extensions

Do-it-yourself, seamless, clip-in extensions blended into waves of soft hair so the extensions look natural and the hair looks full, sexy, and healthy.

other must HAVES

+ Sally Hershberger Brilliant **Hairspray**, $12.50; www.sallyhershberger.com

+ **Small clip-in extensions** for fun moments— ponytail wraps, clip-in bangs, or instant ponytails: POP Put on Pieces, prices vary; www.hairuwear .com

+ **Synthetic extensions** for humid environments, since they don't respond to temperature changes

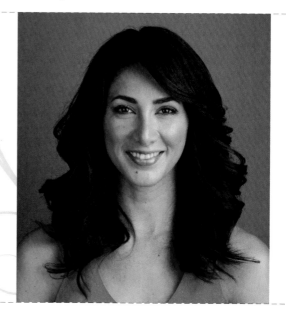

THE SCOOP

Extensions fill in where your normal hair cannot. "Extensions add instant fullness and length around the face and shoulders to give hair more shape," says celebrity stylist Sally Hershberger. Prime candidates for extensions include people who have trouble growing their hair long enough for face-flattering layers and those who don't want to harm their hair by coloring it. And, given their temporary nature, extensions are great for test-driving a new style. "Clip-ins are easy to maintain, are great for short time periods, and can be taken in and out in a snap," she says.

BEST BETS

You need to think about matching your hair color, texture, and length when buying extensions. "Finding quality hair extensions and applying them properly is also important," says Hershberger. Part of the success lies in the technique. "You need to attach enough hair so your real hair and the extensions blend. If they don't, it looks fake." Depending on the quality, real hair extensions can cost anywhere from $100 to $800. Synthetic hair extensions are much more affordable and start at $50. "Avoid purchasing over the Internet," she says. "It's always better to see the hair in person."

APPLY THIS

Where you want to put in the extension, tease the hair at the roots, then spray hairspray for texture and hold. Blow dry to set. Then clip the extensions to the roots where the hair has been teased. This process should take only ten to fifteen minutes. Extensions are even easier to blend and hide with wavy hair. Be careful, though: While human hair extensions can be manipulated with heat tools (flat iron, curling iron, hot rollers, etc.), synthetic extensions will melt.

toss

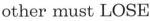

bad extensions

Separated, stringy, poorly placed clip-in extensions that don't blend with the natural hair and look like scarecrow hair poking out haphazardly.

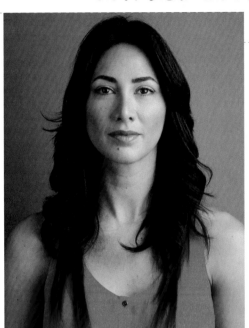

other must LOSE

— Shiny, **high-gloss synthetic extensions** that don't match your hair texture

— **Synthetic extensions** you've had **longer than three months** or **human hair extensions** you've had **more than a year**—this is when they start to degrade

— **Super chunky hairpieces**—like a braided bun—that make your head look top-heavy

ditch it

"At-home extensions look terrible when they are mismatched, stringy, and exposed at the roots," says Hershberger. "They also look fake if the length is way longer than the natural hair."

tricks of the trade

Part of making extensions seamless is concealing and blending them with your natural hair. When you don't properly prep the hair for clip-ins, it just makes them achingly obvious. "Putting them where the hair naturally parts makes them visible and ill-fitting on the head and is the number one mistake women make," says Hershberger.

apply this

Don't leave clip-ins attached overnight. Warns Hershberger, "The teasing can damage the hair."

age alert

As we age, we lose hair. And while nearly all hair types can benefit from extensions, there is one type of person who's out of luck. "If you are older and your hair is thinner, it is hard to keep extensions in," Hershberger says.

wear

undone bun

A low chignon that hits at the base of the neck, has wisps of hair sticking out, and is not pulled back achingly ballerina-tight.

other must HAVES

+ **Tight bun** if you have a round face—it streamlines your look

+ **Relaxed updo** if you have a long face (rounds out features) or curly hair (a romantic silhouette)

+ **Sleek hair**—an easy texture to wind tight

+ Rene Furterer **Styling Wax**, $23; drugstores and mass retailers

THE SCOOP

"*Chignon* is simply French for a low bun," says Nexxus creative director Kevin Mancuso, who has styled updos on Taylor Swift, Natalie Portman, and Sienna Miller.

AGE ALERT

You can wear a bun at any age, but think about placement. A low bun draws eyes directly to your neck and chin and is best worn by women who have a naturally long neck. If your neck is wrinkly, Mancuso suggests wearing the bun high. It brings up the focus to the face, eyes, and cheekbones.

APPLY THIS

For a fun bun with unexpected twists and curls, Mancuso suggests this. Apply a texture-enhancing lotion like Nexxus VersaStyler to damp hair. Flip your head down and blow dry your hair, concentrating on the roots. When the hair is mostly dry, flip back up and use a round brush to smooth out the hair around the face (the back needs the volume, so leave it as is). Rub a styling wax on your hands, use your fingers to rake the hair back into a low, loose ponytail, and secure with an elastic. Loosely twist the ponytail into a coiled donut shape, tucking any loose ends underneath. Secure with bobby pins.

TRICKS OF THE TRADE

For women with fine hair that slips out of updos, Mancuso suggests backcombing and teasing the hair while it's in the ponytail, and applying hairspray before twisting into the bun. "This will help create more texture and body and hold the bun in place," he says.

stylish side pony

A side ponytail of wavy hair and loose wisps that sits on one shoulder, with side-swept bangs.

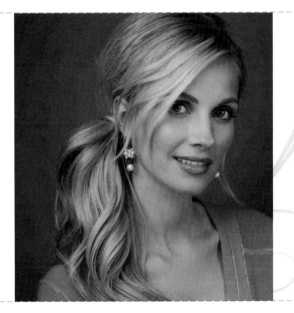

other must HAVES

+ **Volume-enhancing mousse**: Nexxus Mousse Plus ($2.99; www.nexxus.com or drugstores and mass retailers) or Leonor Greyl Voluforme Setting Spray ($34; www.amazon.com)

+ **Silk pillowcase or silk scarf** (to wrap hair while you sleep); silk is gentler and less abrasive than rougher fabrics

+ **Sleekly pulled back, low ponytail** with curly, wavy ends for a modern take

APPLY THIS

Get the perfect side pony by working a volume-enhancing mousse through damp hair from root to tip. Dry hair using a hairdryer with a diffuser to maximize body and bring out natural texture. When dry, separate the top section of the hair and clip it aside, pulling the rest back to create a low side ponytail. Secure with an elastic. Take the top section and spray at the root with a light-hold hairspray like Nexxus Comb Thru to add volume. If you have bangs, pull these out of the top section first. Let them fall naturally around your face. Comb the top section back and wrap the loose ends around the elastic. Use a bobby pin to secure. Finish with a dime-size amount of Nexxus Sleek Finish smoothing cream to control frizz and flyaways. If you have bangs, hairspray sections of hair back toward the ponytail, allowing the shortest pieces to naturally frame your face.

AGE ALERT

"The older the woman, the lower the ponytail should be, and vice versa," warns Mancuso. "A lower ponytail provides a more sophisticated silhouette, whereas a really high ponytail, while chic for some, may read too trendy on a mature woman."

TRICKS OF THE TRADE

Mancuso uses a boar bristle brush that smooths out kinks and bumps when brushing back hair. He cautions that you should never tighten the ponytail by separating the loose ends into two sections and pulling apart—this promotes breakage. And always take a small piece of hair from the ponytail and wrap it around the elastic, securing with a bobby pin. "It is such an easy step, but it instantly refines the ponytail and makes it look polished," he says.

wear this, toss that to win!

We all have that one outfit we run to in a pinch. It fits our body perfectly and never wrinkles. You cherish the fact that you bought it on sale or on consignment or as a splurge, because from the moment you slipped it on, it moved with you. It's the outfit you recycle for different events—date night, book club, or a night out with the girls—because you've already lined up the chic accessories to go with it: cute chandelier earrings, the just-right handbag, and heels that don't hurt.

Why are you repeatedly drawn to this ensemble? Because it is an at-the-ready, grab-and-go no brainer and you feel sensational every time you wear it.

By now you should have a closet full of clothes and a bathroom full of beauty products that you adore and give you the buzz of empowerment. Obliterated is the self-doubt. Gone is the frustration with frumpy. Retired are the clothes that did nothing for you but weigh you down and bum you out physically *and* emotionally.

You deserve this newfound feeling of fabulousness and clarity because you've worked hard to achieve it. Fashion can be nonsensical until you define it in a way that makes sense to you, and this is precisely what I've tried to do with **WEAR THIS, TOSS THAT!**

Now that we are ending our time together, my parting pages highlight our models wearing some farewell looks, the invaluable **save-me**'s found throughout the book, and hundreds of web sites, retailers, and brands for savvy shopping. I wish I could guarantee that bad fashion days are forever a thing of the past, but fashion is fluid. In jumping in midstream, we're bound, occasionally, to miss our footing. But that's part of the trip. That's what makes this journey such a thrill. Break your own rules. Make your own splash. And promise, no matter what, to make your look *your signature own.*

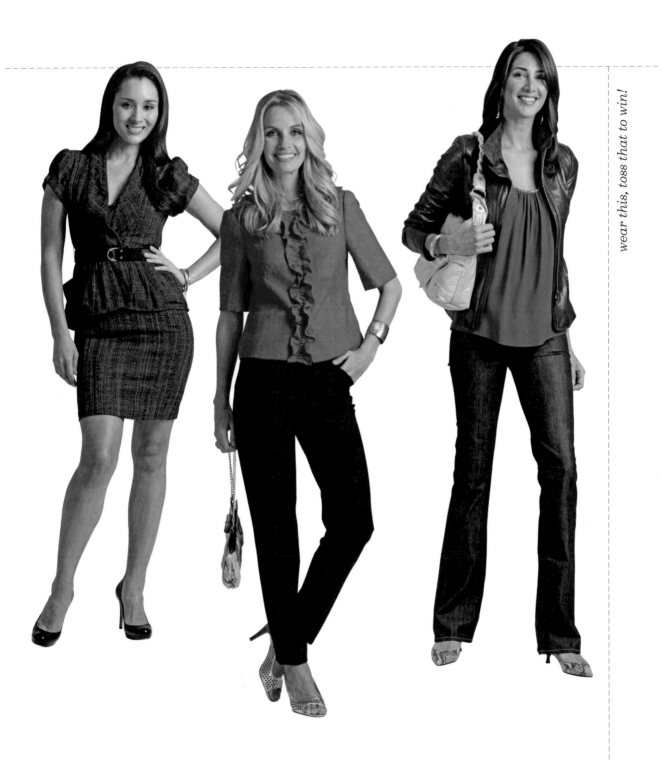

189

my 24 **save-me's** that will keep you fashionably afloat

1. **WRAP SHIRT:** These shirts do double duty, showing off skin while hiding bulk. Back and side ties both make for attractive accoutrements…page 6

2. **BOOB TUBE:** Avoid wardrobe malfunctions with the Boob Tube by Miss Oops. The lace bandeau covers your chest without adding visual pounds…page 6

3. **THE LAUNDRESS WOOL & CASHMERE SHAMPOO:** Get your sweaters super soft with this shampoo; it's cheaper than dry cleaning and good for the environment, too…page 17

4. **SEXY KNIT:** Whether you choose a sexy draped style or something more tailored, make sure to pick a knit with interesting detail, like sparkles or an exciting color…page 20

5. **SOMA INTIMATES VANISHING EDGE PANTIES:** Rejoice, because you'll never have VPL (visible panty lines) again with these undies, which are the ultimate in comfort. They're available in boyshort, brief, bikini, and hipster…page 28

6. **BRISTOLS 6 HEM TAPE FOR DENIM:** Make your jeans more versatile with this hem tape, which allows you to hike your jeans up temporarily, whether you're wearing modest peep-toe pumps or sky-high stilettos…page 36

7. **DARK DENIM WIDE-LEGGED TROUSERS:** If you like to wear denim but want to keep it classy in the office, try pairing these trousers with a cute blouse or sweater and pumps…page 36

8. **SPANX TIGHT-END TIGHTS:** Mix it up and slim your legs at the same time with patterned, textured, and printed tights from Spanx…page 48

9. **A-LINE DRESS:** This dress is great for all body types—if you have hips, the dress's fitted bodice and lower half smoothes over them, while if you're boy-straight, it will give you the illusion of curves…page 60

10. **METALLIC SHRUG:** Don't even think about pairing that dress with a matching jacket or wrap—boring! Instead, mix up your formalwear with a metallic shrug. It goes with pretty much everything…page 65

11. **SHIRTS TO GO UNDER YOUR SUIT JACKETS:** It's tough remembering which shirt goes with which jacket. That's why I've done the work for you, grouping my pairings in a handy chart so you'll always look well suited whether you're at a board meeting or a job interview…page 73

12. **VAUTE COUTURE:** If you like the look of leather but aren't into the whole "wearing animals" thing, try Vaute Couture for some seriously amazing vegan coats…page 81

13. **FOOTZY ROLLS:** When your tootsies are tired, grab a pair of Footzy Rolls— rollable ballet flats that hide in your purse until you need them. Your feet will thank you!...page 89

14. **T-STRAP SHOE:** The T-strap is versatile—it narrows a wider foot by breaking up the foot's expanse down the middle, and it widens a narrow foot by lending width with the strap...page 90

15. **UNDER THE KNEE BOOT:** Slide these on with just about anything and see how they magically slim your calves...page 94

16. **REMOVABLE HEEL PROTECTOR:** Everyday walking takes a toll on your shoes. Avoid broken heels (and broken hearts!) with the Smart Heel...page 96

17. **PAIN-FREE FOOTWEAR:** Who says you can't be stylish and comfortable at the same time? I've found the best brands in the biz, which use the latest technology to keep your feet comfy and fashionable, and collected them in this chart for you ...page 99

18. **MEDIUM-WIDTH BELT:** All body types can rock this cincher, which is generally one to two inches wide. Wear it a bit above your natural waistline for a super trendy look...page 112

19. **EMBELLISHED BELT:** Not only are these belts totally in the moment, they're also great for minimizing hips. Cinch at the waist and your eyes will move to your upper body and away from the hips...page 118

20. **CHANDELIER EARRINGS:** These elegant danglers are so versatile that you can wear them with any outfit, dressy or casual. Chandelier earrings set off most face shapes. Long faces should steer clear, though, as they further extend...page 123

21. **BANGLE:** Whether it's silver, gold, embellished, or studded, the bangle pairs well with almost any other piece of jewelry and is an absolute essential to own...page 126

22. **SHISEIDO TOTAL REVITALIZING CREAM:** From its new Future Solution LX line, Shiseido has created a moisturizer that will leave you with velvety soft skin. A technology called Skingencell 1P helps promote healthier, more resilient skin cells. At just under $100, it's not exactly cheap, but a little will last you a long time...page 136

23. **POWDER BLUSH:** It's easier to apply than cream, and you can achieve more vivid color with powder blush. Powder is especially beneficial for oily skin because it absorbs excess oil, but it works well with all skin types...page 150

24. **DRY SHAMPOO:** Apply to scalp to absorb oil between shampooing and make hair look and smell fresh without having to jump in the shower...page 171

savvy shopping

1 top rack: shirts & sweaters

Ann Taylor, www.anntaylor.com or 800-DIAL-ANN

Bluefly, www.bluefly.com or 877-BLUEFLY

Boutique to You, www.boutiquetoyou.com

Brooks Brothers, www.brooksbrothers.com or 800-274-1815

Claudia Lobao jewelry, www.claudialobao.com for info, www.shoprumor.com

Covet Shop, www.covetshop.com or 212-228-0648

eBay, www.ebay.com

Ella Moss, www.ellamoss.com or 866-290-1384

ELLE, www.kohls.com

Emporio Armani, www.emporioarmani.com or 866-602-7799

Etsy, www.etsy.com or www.deniz03.etsy.com

H&M, www.hm.com/us for stores

Joie, www.joie.com for stores, or Bloomingdale's

Jovovich Hawk, www.jovovichhawk.com

The Laundress, www.thelaundress.com

LC Lauren Conrad, www.kohls.com

Love21 Contemporary, www.forever21.com or 888-494-3837

M&J Trimming, www.mjtrim.com or 800-9-MJTRIM

Maidenform, www.maidenform.com or 888-888-9328

Miss Oops, www.missoops.com

Mod Cloth, www.modcloth.com or 888-495-9699

Newport News, www.newport-news.com or 800-688-2830

Precision Hangers, www.precisionhangers.com or 212-967-3177

Proenza Schonler, www.proenzaschonler.com

Ralph Lauren Rugby, www.rugby.com or 866-99-RUGBY

Romeo & Juliet Couture, www.romeoandjulietcouture.com

Rusty Zipper, www.rustyzipper.com or 866-387-5944

Second Time Around, www.secondtimearound.net

Shapeez, www.unblievabra.com or 877-360-8426

Shop It To Me, www.shopittome.com

Shopstyle, www.shopstyle.com

The Snob, www.thesnob.net or 877-590-SNOB

Stella McCartney, www.stellamccartney.com

Strap Doctor, www.strapdoctor.com

Swap Ace, www.swapace.com

Sweetees, www.mellies.com for info, www.shopstyle.com

Target, www.target.com or 800-591-3869

Top Shop, www.us.topshop.com or 866-853-8559

Tres Sleek, www.tressleek.com or 800-471-3830

Uniqlo, www.uniqlo.com or 877-4-UNIQLO

Wacoal, www.wacoal-america.com for stores

2 bottom rack: pants & skirts

Anthropologie, www.anthropologie.com or 800-309-2500

Banana Republic, www.bananarepublic.com or 888-277-8953

Bisou Bisou for JCPenney, www.jcp.com or 800-322-1189

Bluefly, www.bluefly.com or 877-BLUEFLY

Bristols 6, www.bristols6.com

Citizens of Humanity, www.citizensofhumanity.com for stores

CJ by Cookie Johnson, www.cjbycookiejohnson.com or www.nordstrom.com/cjcookiejohnson.com

Commandos, www.gocommandos.com or 866-970-FREE

Ebates, www.ebates.com

Fashion-Fix by Topstick, www.vapon.com or 800-443-8856

Free Shipping, www.freeshipping.org

Gap, www.gap.com or 800-427-7895

Gilt Fuse, www.giltfuse.com

Gilt Group, www.gilt.com

Hudson, www.hudsonjeans.com

Hue, www.hue.com or 800-575-3497

Isaac Mizrahi for Liz Claiborne, www.lcnyoutlet.com

J Brand, www.jbrandjeans.com

JCPenney, www.jcp.com

JOE's Jeans, www.joesjeans.com or 877-413-7467

Jones New York, www.jny.com or 888-255-7992

K-mart, www.kmart.com

Levi Strauss & Co., www.levi.com or 866-860-8907

Lucky Brand, www.luckybrand.com or 866-975-5825

Marc Jacobs, www.marcjacobs.com or 877-707-6272

Miss Oops, www.missoops.com

My True Fit, www.mytruefit.com or 877-FIT-TRUE

Nicole by Nicole Miller at JCPenney, www.jcp.com or 800-322-1189

Paige Premium Denim, www.paigepremiumdenim.com or www.paigeusa.com

Relic NY, www.relicny.com

Rent the Runway, www.renttherun way.com or 800-509-0842

Retail Me Not, www.retailmenot.com

Serfontaine, www.serfontaine.com

7 For All Mankind, www.7forallmankind.com or 866-427-1114

Simply Vera Vera Wang, www.kohls .com

Soma Intimates, www.soma.com or 866-768-7662

Spanx, www.spanx.com or 800-806-7311

True Religion Brand Jeans, www.truereligionbrandjeans.com or 866-427-1119

Wal-mart, www.walmart.com or 800-WALMART

Wolford, www.wolford.com or 800-WOLFORD

Xhilaration by Target, www.target .com or 800-591-3869

3 hanging rack: dresses, suits, & coats

Aerosoles, www.aerosoles.com or 800-798-9478

Albert Nipon, available at www.neimanmarcus.com

Amazon, www.amazon.com or 866-216-1072

Armani, www.giorgioarmani.com

Badgley Mischka, Badgley Mischka Platinum Label, and Mark + James, www.badgleymischka.com

Bare Necessities, www.bare necessities.com or 877-728-9272

BCBG Max Azria, www.bcbg.com

Bebe, www.bebe.com

Billion Dollar Babes, www.billion dollarbabes.com or 888-300-6254

Bottomless Closet, www.bottomless closet.org

Bring It Up, www.bringitup.com or 800-670-6201

Burberry, www.us.burberry.com or 800-284-8480

Calvin Klein, www.calvinklein.com or 866-513-0513

Carmen Marc Valvo, www.carmen marcvalvo.com or 800-4-CARMEN

Charlotte Russe, www.charlotterusse .com

The Dessy Group, www.dessy.com

DKNY, www.dkny.com

Dress for Success, www.dressfor success.org or 212-532-1922

Edition by Erin Fetherston, www.qvc.com or 888-345-5788

Edressme, www.edressme.com or 866-433-7377

Elie Tahari, www.elietahari.com or 800-545-0799

Erin Fetherston, www.erinfetherston .com or 212-643-7537

Ever, www.ever-us.com

Express, www.express.com or 888-397-1980

Farinaz Taghavi, www.farinaz.com

Fiebing, www.fiebing.com or 800-558-1033

1st Dibs, www.1stdibs.com

Gap, www.gap.com or 800-427-7895

Ideeli, www.ideeli.com

J.Crew, www.jcrew.com or 800-562-0258

Jones New York, www.jny.com

Katy Beh, www.katybeh.com or 877-KATYBEH

Kenneth Cole, www.kennethcole.com or 800-KEN-COLE

La Rok, www.larok.com

Lauren by Ralph Lauren, www.ralphlauren.com or 888-475-7674

Loehmann's, www.loehmanns.com or 800-366-5634

London Fog, www.londonfog.com or 800-413-9133

Mango, www.mangoshop.com or 866-666-4664

Michael Kors, www.michaelkors.com or 800-908-1157

Mint by Jodi Arnold, www.jodiarnold nyc.com or 347-270-8610

Miss Me Collection, www.missme .com or 877-600-7351

Miu Miu, www.miumiu.com or 212-641-2980

Net-A-Porter, www.net-a-porter.com or 800-481-1064

Nine West, www.ninewest.com or 800-999-1877

The North Face, www.thenorthface .com or 888-TNF-1968

The Outnet, www.theoutnet.com or 866-785-8246

Rebecca Taylor, www.rebeccataylor .com or 212-966-0406

Reverse Reverse, www.reverse-reverse.com

Revolveclothing, www.revolve clothing.com or 888-442-5830

Screaming Mimi's, www.screaming mimis.com or 212-677-6464

Shop Intuition, www.shopintuition .com

Shop It To Me, www.shopittome.com

Shop It Up Chic, www.shopitup chic.com

Shop Style, www.shopstyle.com

Simply Vera, www.kohls.com or 866-887-8884

Soma Intimates, www.soma.com or 866-768-7662

Spanx, www.spanx.com or 800-806-7311

Stefani Greenfield's Curations, www.hsn.com or 800-284-5757

Thakoon, www.thakoon.com

Theory, www.theory.com or 877-242-3317

Thread Lounge, www.threadlounge .com or 415-503-1437/415-717-3957 in San Francisco, 773-281-0011 in Chicago

Top Shop, www.topshop.com or 866-853-8559

Tracy Reese, www.tracyreese.com

Urban Outfitters, www.urban outfitters.com or 800-959-8794

Vaute Couture, www.vautecouture.com

Vegetarian Shoes, www.vegetarian-shoes.co.uk or +44(0)1273 691913

Vera Wang, www.verawang.com

Vince, www.vince.com or 800-960-2231

Vivienne Tam, www.viviennetam.com or 212-966-2398

Wasteland Clothing, www.wasteland clothing.com

Yummie Tummie, www.yummie tummie.com or 402-935-2050

Zara, www.zara.com

4 shoe rack

Aerosoles, www.aerosoles.com

Anyi Lu, www.anyilu.com

Cole Haan Air, www.colehaan.com or 800-695-8945

DKNY Donna Karan New York, www.dkny.com or 888-521-2819

Donald J. Pliner, www.donaldjpliner.com or 888-307-1630

Endless, www.endless.com or 866-218-9936

Elizabeth and James, www.elizabeth andjames.us or 212-382-1780

Footzy Rolls, www.footzyrolls.com

Hunter, www.hunter-boot.com or 877-495-1500

Hush Puppies, www.hushpuppies.com or 866-699-7365

Jessica Simpson Collection, www.jessicasimpsoncollection.com

Kenneth Cole 925, www.kennethcole.com or 800-KEN-COLE

LiftKits, www.myliftkits.com

Mia, www.miashoes.com

Milk & Honey, www.milkandhoney shoes.com

Nine West, www.ninewest.com or 800-999-1877

Payless Shoes, www.payless.com or 877-474-6379

Piperlime, www.piperlime.com or 877-PIPERLIME

PolarWrap, www.polarwrap.com or 800-967-WRAP

Pour La Victoire, www.pourlavictoire.com or 212-460-8000

Restricted Shoes, www.restricted shoes.com or 626-961-8889

Seychelles, www.seychellesfootwear.com or 800-453-3077

Shoe Angels, www.myshoeangels.com

Shoebuy, www.shoebuy.com or 888-200-8414

Shoebuy designer division, www.designer.shoebuy.com or 888-200-8414

Silhouettes, www.silhouettes.com or 888-651-8337

SmartHeel, www.smartheel.com

Target, www.target.com or 800-591-3869

Taryn Rose, www.tarynrose.com or 877-404-ROSE

Zappos, www.zappos.com

5 top shelf: handbags

Barneys, www.barneys.com

Coach, www.coach.com

eFashion House, www.efashion house.com

Endless, www.endless.com

Etsy, www.etsy.com

Fashionphile, www.fashionphile.com

Hayden Harnett, haydenharnett.com

Laudividini, www.laudividini.com

Lauren Merkin, www.laurenmerkin.com

Lexol Leather Care, www.lexol.com

LuxeLink, www.luxelink.com

Matt & Nat, www.mattandnat.com

My Theresa, www.mytheresa.com

Neiman Marcus, www.neiman marcus.com

Net-a-porter, www.net-a-porter.com

Pursendipity, www.pursendipity.net

Revival Boutique, www.revival boutique.com

Rue La La, www.ruelala.com

Saks Fifth Avenue, www.saksfifth avenue.com

Target, www.target.com

Vintage Instyle, www.vintage-instyle.com

What Goes Around Comes Around, www.whatgoesaroundnyc.com

Zappos, couture.zappos.com

6 accessory drawer: belts

B-Low The Belt, www.b-lowthebelt.com

Bluefly, www.bluefly.com or 877-BLUEFLY

Calvin Klein, www.calvinklein.com or 866-513-0513

Elegantly Waisted, www.shopbop.com or 877-SHOPBOP

Kristin Kahle, www.kristinkahle.com or 858-412-5861

Ralph Lauren, www.ralphlauren.com or 888-475-7674

7 accessory box: jewelry

All The Rage Online, www.allthe rageonline.com or 888-509-8088

Anna Sheffield for Target, www.target.com

Barneys New York, www.barneys.com

Bee Charming, www.bcharming.net

Bloomingdale's, www.bloomingdales.com or 800-777-0000

Carol Brodie, Rarities, HSN, www.hsn.com or 800-284-5757

Carolee, www.carolee.com or 800-227-6533

Edition by Banana Republic, www.bananarepublic.gap.com or 800-427-7895

Etsy, www.etsy.com

Fragments, www.fragments.com or 866-966-4688

Giving Tree Jewelry, www.givingtree jewelry.com or 888-246-3551

Hollywood Intuition by Jaye Hersh for Target, www.target.com or 800-591-3869

J.Crew, www.jcrew.com or 800-562-0258

Laura James Jewelry, www.laura jamesjewelry.com

Max & Chloe, www.maxandchloe.com or 646-290-6446

Molly Sims, Grayce, HSN, www.hsn .com or 800-284-5757

Moondance Jewelry Gallery, www.moondancejewelry.com or 877-EST-1989

New Twist, www.newtwist.com

Nicole Miller, www.nicolemiller.com or 888-300-6258

Satya Jewelry, www.satyajewelry.com or 877-728-9269

Shop The Look, www.shopthelook.net or 347-227-4650

Three Sisters Jewelry Design by Zoe, www.threesistersjewelrydesign .com

Timex, www.timex.com, www.timex stylewatch.com, or 800-448-4639

Tina Tang Jewelry, www.tinatang.com or 212-645-6890

8 skincare shelf

AHAVA, www.ahavaus.com

Aveeno, www.aveeno.com

Bare Escentuals, www.bare escentuals.com or 888-795-4747

Barielle, www.barielle.com or 800-790-8884

Beauty Blitz, www.beautyblitz.com

Bioré, www.bonanzle.com or www.ebay.com

The Body Shop, www.thebody shop-usa.com

Bonanzle, www.bonanzle.com

Boots, www.target.com or www.us.boots.com

Borba, www.borba.com

Burt's Bees, www.burtsbees.com or 800-849-7112

C.O. Bigelow, www.bigelowchemists .com

Cetaphil, www.cetaphil.com

Chantecaille, www.chantecaille.com

Chapstick, www.chapstick.com or www.drugstore.com

Clarins, www.usclarins.com

Clearasil, www.clearasil.us, www.homesolutionsstore.com, or 800-820-8939

CVS/Pharmacy, www.cvs.com

DERMAdoctor, www.dermadoctor .com

Dior, www.dior.com or 866-503-9490

Dove, www.dove.com

Dr. Brandt, www.drbrandtskincare.com

Dr. Hauschka, www.drhauschka.com

Drugstore.com, www.drugstore.com

eBay, www.ebay.com

Elizabeth Arden Prevage, www.prevageskin.com

Estée Lauder, www.esteelauder.com

Evian, www.amazon.com

Fresh, www.fresh.com

Garnier, www.garnier.com

H20+, www.h20plus.com or 800-242-2284

Josie Maran, www.josiemaran.com

Kate Somerville, www.katesomerville .com

Kiehl's, www.kiehls.com

Kinerase, www.kinerase.com

La Roche-Posay, www.laroche-posay .us

Lancome, www.lancome-usa.com

Laura Geller, www.laurageller.com

LipCotz, www.amazon.com

Lumene, www.cvs.com

LypSyl, www.lypsylhome.com

Macy's, www.macys.com

Mary Kay, www.marykay.com

MD Formulations, www.bare escentuals.com

Muji, www.muji.us

Murad, www.murad.com or 800-33-MURAD

Neiman Marcus, www.neimanmarcus .com or 888-888-4757

Neutrogena, www.neutrogena.com

Nia24, www.nia24.com

Nordstrom, www.nordstrom.com

Nude Skincare, www.nudeskincare .com

Olay, www.olay.com

100 Percent Pure Organic, www.100percentpure.com

The Organic Pharmacy, www.the organicpharmacy.com

Peter Thomas Roth, www.peter thomasroth.com

REN, www.renskincare.com or www.drugstore.com

RoC, www.rocskincare.com

St. Ives, www.stives.com

Shiseido, www.sca.shiseido.com

SkinMedica, www.skinmedica.com

Target, www.target.com

Tarte Cosmetics, www.tarte cosmetics.com

Total Block, www.dermadoctor.com

Ulta Beauty, www.ulta.com

Vanicream, www.psico.com for info, or www.drugstore.com

Yu-Be, www.amazon.com

Walgreens, www.walgreens.com

9 cosmetics drawer

Alba, www.albabotanica.com

Almay, www.almay.com

Amazon, www.amazon.com

Anastasia, www.anastasia.net

Ardell Fashion Lashes, www.ardelllashes.com

Bare Essentials, www.bareessentials.com

bareMinerals, www.bareescentuals.com

BeautyBlender, www.beautyblender.net

Beauty.com, www.beauty.com

beautyblitz, www.beautyblitz.com

Becca Cosmetics, www.beccacosmetics.com

Benefit, www.benefitcosmetics.com

Bergdorf Goodman, www.bergdorfgoodman.com

Black Opal, www.blackopalbeauty.com

Bloomingdale's, www.bloomingdales.com or 800-777-0000

Bobbi Brown, www.bobbibrowncosmetics.com

Boots No7, www.us.boots.com, www.target.com, or 800-591-3869

Brush Off, www.brushoff.com

Burt's Bees, www.burtsbees.com

Buxom, www.bareescentuals.com

Cargo, www.cargocosmetics.com

Chanel, www.chanel.com or 800-550-0005

Clarins, www.us.clarins.com

Cle de Peu Beauté, www.cledepeau-beaute.com

Clean & Clear, www.cleanandclear.com

CoverGirl, www.covergirl.com

CVS Beauty 360, www.cvs.com

Dillards, www.dillards.com

Dior, www.dior.com or 866-503-9490

Drugstore.com, www.drugstore.com

Duo, www.drugstore.com

DuWop, www.shop.duwop.com

e.l.f., www.eyeslipsface.com

Essence of Beauty, CVS, www.cvs.com

Estée Lauder, www.esteelauder.com

Eve Pearl, www.evepearl.com

Face, www.sephora.com

Giorgio Armani, www.giorgioarmanibeauty.com

Global Goddess, www.globalgoddessbeauty.com

Guerlain, www.guerlain.com

Hard Candy, www.hardcandy.com

Haute Look, www.hautelook.com

It Cosmetics, www.itcosmetics.com

Iman Cosmetics, www.imancosmetics.com

Japonesque, www.japonesque.com

Jordana, www.jordanacosmetics.com

Josie Maran, www.josiemaran.com

Kevyn Aucoin, www.kevynaucoindirect.com or 866-541-7382

L'Oréal Paris, www.loreal.com

Laura Geller, www.laurageller.com

Laura Mercier, www.lauramercier.com

Le Métier de Beauté, www.metierbeaute.com

Leslie Marnett, www.beautydean.com

MAC Cosmetics, www.maccosmetics.com or 800-588-0070

Mally Beauty, www.mallybeauty.com

Maybelline New York, www.maybelline.com or www.drugstore.com

NARS, www.narscosmetics.com

Nick Barose, www.nickbarose.com

Nordstrom, www.nordstrom.com

100 Percent Pure Organic, www.100percentpure.com

Organic Wear, www.physiciansformula.com or www.beauty.com

Philosophy, www.philosophy.com

Physicians Formula, www.physiciansformula.com

POP Beauty, www.popbeauty.co.uk

Pür Minerals, www.purminerals.com

QVC, www.qvc.com

Revlon, www.revlon.com

Saks Fifth Avenue, www.saksfifthavenue.com

Sephora, www.sephora.com or 877-SEPHORA

Shiseido, www.sca.shiseido.com

Shu Uemura, www.shuuemura-usa.com

Smashbox, www.smashbox.com or 888-763-1361

Sonia Kashuk, www.target.com

Stila, www.stilacosmetics.com

Target, www.target.com

Tarte, www.tartecosmetics.com

Three Custom Color Specialists, www.threecustom.com

Tweezerman, www.tweezerman.com

Ulta Beauty, www.ulta.com

Urban Decay, www.urbandecay.com

Walgreens, www.walgreens.com

Wal-mart, www.walmart.com

Wet n Wild, www.wnwbeauty.com

Yves Saint Laurent, www.yslbeautyus.com

10 haircare shelf

Alberto V05, www.drugstore.com

Arturo of Arturo New York, www.houseofarturo.com

Amazon, www.amazon.com

Aveeno, www.aveeno.com

BaByliss, www.babylisspro.co.uk or www.folica.com

Beauty Ticket, www.beautyticket.com

Beautypedia, www.beautypedia.com

Bergdorf Goodman, www.bergdorfgoodman.com

Bumble and Bumble, www.bumbleandbumble.com

Charles Worthington, www.charlesworthington.com

Chi USA, www.chiretail.com or www.amazon.com

Conair, www.conair.com

Denman, www.denmanbrush.com

Enzo Milano, www.shopenzomilano.com

Folica, www.folica.com

Frederic Fekkai, www.fekkai.com

Garnier Fructis, www.garnier.com

ghd, www.ghdhair.com/us

Hercut, www.hercut.com or www.sephora.com

Hot Tools, www.folica.com

HSN, www.hsn.com

John Frieda, www.johnfrieda.com

Joico, www.joico.com

Kérastase, www.keratase-usa.com

Kevin Mancuso, celebrity hair stylist and Nexxus creative director, www.kevinmancuso.com

Komenuka Bijin, www.komenuka-bijin.com or 877-737-4247

Kronos, www.kronoshair.com

Leonor Greyl, www.leonorgreyl.com or www.amazon.com

Locks of Love, www.locksoflove.org

L'Oréal Paris, www.loreal.com

Lucky, www.jatai.net > products > lucky grip clips

Marilyn Brushes, www.marilynbrush.com

Mason Pearson, www.masonpearson.com

Mizani, www.mizani-usa.com

MoroccanOil, www.moroccanoil.com or fine salons

Naturia by Rene Furerer, www.sephora.com

Neimann Marcus, www.neimannmarcus.com

Neutrogena, www.neutrogena.com

Nexxus, www.nexxus.com

Oscar Blandi, www.sephora.com

Ouidad, www.ouidad.com

Pantene, www.pantene.com

Paula Begoun, www.beautypedia.com

Paul Mitchell, www.paulmitchell.com or Paul Mitchell salons

Phyto, www.phyto-usa.com or 800-55-PHYTO

POP Put on Pieces, www.hairuwear.com

Rene Furterer, www.renefurterer.com or www.sephora.com

Sally Hershberger, www.sallyhershberger.com

Sephora, www.sephora.com

Shu Uemura, www.shuuemuraartofhair-usa.com

Solano, www.solanopower.com or 800-323-3942

Spornette, www.spornette.com

Ted Gibson, www.tedgibsonsalon.com

Tigi Bed Head, www.tigihaircare.com

Total Beauty, www.totalbeauty.com

T3 Bespoke Labs, www.t3micro.com

photo credits

All photography by Stephen Sullivan, except for the following:

vi Amy Goodman
Anna Moller, www.annamoller.net

xviii Tatum clutch
Lauren Merkin

52 trumpet skirt
Anthropologie

53 lace/ruffled skirt
Tracy Reese

90 slingback
Via Spiga

91 wedge
Stuart Weitzman

92 pointy toe flat
Via Spiga

93 flip flop
Carlos by Carlos Santana

94 under the knee boot
Via Spiga

95 rocker/biker boot
Stuart Weitzman

97 thong
Sperry Topsider

98 espadrille
Butter

105 pochette
iStockphoto/ © Albert Smirnov

118 jeweled belt
B-low the Belt

140 4-in-1 Cleansing Treatment
Scott-Vincent Borba

151 Chanel Le Sourcil De Chanel Perfect Brows
courtesy of CHANEL

158 Chanel Rouge Coco Hydrating Crème Lip Colour
courtesy of CHANEL

162 Anastasia Beverly Hills Brow Tool Kit
Anastasia Beverly Hills

172 Nexxus Salon Hair Care Lavish Body, Thermal Volume
Nexxus

fashion credits

contents

1 top rack: shirts & sweaters

2 bottom rack: pants & skirts

93 casual flats
loafer flat by Sperry Top-Sider
flip flop by Carlos by Carlos Santana
fashion sneaker by Geox

94 boots
under the knee by Via Spiga
mid-calf at Endless.com
ankle/peep toe by Stuart Weitzman
over the knee at ShoptheShoeBox.com

95
rocker/biker by Stuart Weitzman
equestrian/riding at ShoptheShoeBox.com
western by Frye

96 sandals
super strappy by Spring
wooden by Seychelles
metallic slingback at T.J.Maxx

97
thong by Sperry Topsider
gladiator by Via Spiga

98 ethnic
clog by Born
moccasin by Sofft
espadrille by Butter

5 top shelf: handbags

102 bags of ideal size and shape for tall women
sac by Jenny Bird
medium to large unstructured shoulder bag by B. Makowsky
ruffle satchel at Endless.com
handheld clutch by Clara Casavina

104 bags of ideal size and shape for petite women
baguette with strap by Vieta
small shoulder bag by Carlos by Carlos Santana
hobo by Elliott Lucca
bucket bag by Elliott Lucca
small to medium handheld briefcase by Tumi

106 bags of ideal size and shape for tall women
structured, framed satchel by Rebecca Minkoff
square or rectangular shoulder bag by LE'BULGA
tote by LE'BULGA
wristlet by Ada Handbags
oversized envelope or foldover clutch by Dareen Hakim

6 accessory drawer: belts

112 wear leather belt
leather belt by Beltsville
red dress by Lord & Taylor

114 wear skinny metallic belt
skinny metallic belt by Beltsville
purple blouse by Kara Janx

116 wear double buckle belt
double buckle belt by Beltsville
gold dress by Yoana Baraschi

118 wear jeweled belt
jeweled belt by B-low the Belt

7 accessory box: jewelry

122 wear chandelier earrings
rose pearl chandeliers (top left on stand) by Fantasy Jewelry Box at fantasyjewelrybox.com
gold chain drop chandeliers with dark blue crystal beads (top right on stand) by Nashelle
clover chandeliers with rose stones (center on stand) by Vale Jewelry
dark blue crystal chandeliers (bottom left) by Martine Wester
clear crystal chandeliers (bottom right) by Clara Casavina

123 wear stud earrings
all studs by Fantasy Jewelry Box at fantasyjewelrybox.com

124 wear statement necklace
clear rhinestone link necklace by Martine Wester
multi-colored rhinestone necklace with bows by Vale Jewelry
pear-shaped clear rhinestone necklace with gold chain by Fantasy Jewelry Box at fantasyjewelrybox.com

126 wear bangle bracelets
blue crystal bangle by Sorrelli
wooden bangles by Fantasy Jewelry Box at fantasyjewelrybox.com
textured gold bangle by Clara Kasavina

128 wear dress watches
dress bracelet collection watch, gold by Timex
dress crystals collection watch with Swarovski crystals, pink face by Timex
dress crystals collection watch with Swarovski crystals, leather band by Timex

11 wear this, toss that to win!

188
(left) feminine suit by Nanette Lepore at Lord & Taylor
blouse at National Jean Company
bangles by Daniel Espinosa
pumps by Nine West
(center) ruffled jacket by Limited
trousers by Theory at Bloomingdale's
pumps by Franco Sarto
clutch by Elaine Turner
(right) leather jacket by S&K
tank by Kara Janx
jeans by 7 For All Mankind
kitten heels by Stuart Weitzman
tote at Marshall's

acknowledgments

This began as a writer's dream: an out-of-blue telephone call from Judy Linden, who had an idea for a book and wanted me to pen it. Her dedication, sharp editing, and incredibly thoughtful support made these pages happen.

My hat is off to the rest of The Stonesong Press, including the incredibly calm and efficacious Ellen Scordato, who created a shoot and production schedule with superhuman powers, the über-organized and sweet Katherine Latshaw, and the ever-kind Alison Fargis. How lucky was I to land at Atria Books of Simon & Schuster, with Publisher Judith Curr and wonderful Senior Editor Greer Hendricks? Thanks to Sarah Cantin for all of her assistance. And, I doubt anyone outside of family and friends would have heard about this book were it not for Lisa Sciambra and the amazing wonderwoman Amanda Potters.

The talents and speed of photographer Stephen Sullivan made a seemingly impossible shoot schedule fly. To him I take a bow and say, 'NEXT!' (Thanks to Jennifer Crane for the introduction.) I had the great fortune of finding both true beauty and kindness in models Carlota Sosa, Cecilia T., and April Wilkner. And to the fabulous stylist Alana Kelen and her right hand Tal Kohen—may your hard work in pulling clothes solve thousands of fashion dilemmas: a million *mercis* for your tireless efforts and bright smiles.

Grateful, am I, in photographer Gabrielle Revere's artistic eye for my cover shoot and her ability to make me feel beautiful when I was only four months post-partum. Deborah Altizio, thank you for your magic touch. And speaking of magic, designer Alison Lew, your thousands of changes in merging text with images resulted in a magnificent, eye-popping page turner.

I'm fortunate to have every girl's beautification dream team in Arturo and Leslie Marnett. We've been together since the beginning (and survived some beyond early call times) and I'm so proud to call you friends. To the other experts, who carved time into busy schedules to provide valuable insights for this book, I am indebted: Paige Adams-Geller, Sara Blakely, Lauren Merkin, Kate Somerville, Dr. Audrey Kunin, Dr. Fredric Brandt, Scott-Vincent Borba, Mally Roncal, Sara Strand, Nick Barose, Paula Begoun, Sally Hershberger, and Kevin Manucso. And to their publicists who helped marry our schedules: Marina Morrison Keller, Allie Geller, Maggie Adams and

Misty Elliott, Jamie Burnes, Tracy O'Conner, Laura Coppolino, Tara Yamaoka, Brianne Carmody and Niki Turkington, Cynthia Short, Megan Hardwick, and Jacqueline Warren.

Kristine Lumpinski, it was your through-the-grapevine introduction (*merci* Farrah Linden!) that made this happen. To the rest of team Timex…Adam Gurian, Karen Lavin, Corrine Beers of Timex and Liz Kaplow, Shannon Eis, Amelia Woltering, Jeremy Berger, and Juliana Jacobs of Kaplow PR, thank you for making me a part of the family.

I don't believe you arrive in writing a book without mentors and inspirational people who light your path. Martha Nelson, you saw something in me I didn't see in myself and thus began the TV career. Clare McHugh, it has been an honor working for and learning from you all of these years. Jennifer Zawadzinski for your enthusiastic championing in every way. Hal Rubenstein and Cindy Webber-Cleary for the continued inspiration of *In Style*'s fashion pages. America's Junior Miss, a scholarship program (now Distinguished Young Women) for teaching a then teenage girl how to dream big, and then bigger. Grandma Peggy, now 88, for those early lessons on how to dress like a lady.

While writing I said I was giving birth to a book and a baby, the latter my second child born just after the text was due. I didn't survive either process without the gracious support of my extraordinarily patient husband, Michael Lin, who weathered five months of my nightly writing sessions and several months thereafter of my burning the midnight oil. A heartfelt note to the loving grandmothers Mary Ann Goodman and Aio Lin, for traveling far to care for Fi and Ro while I worked. To my dad Dr. George Goodman and father-in-law Dr. Maubee Lin—for living without your wives during their respective visits. My friends, you know who you are, I'm so lucky to have you cheer me on in this crazy ride we call my life.

In becoming a parent, I realize fully the selflessness of my own. Thank you Mom and Dad for your life lessons of compassion, perseverance, and above all, trueness—to who I am and what I do.

resources referred to in this book

Accessories Magazine, www.accessoriesmagazine.com

American Orthopaedic Foot and Ankle Society, www.aofas.org

American Podiatric Medical Association, www.apma.org

Cotton Inc. Lifestyle Monitor, www.lifestylemonitor.cottoninc.com

Bryan Meehan, www.nudeskincare.com

Debenhams, www.debenhams.com

Gamma Beauty Study, www.gammawomen.com

Global Solar UV Index, World Health Organization,
www.who.int/uv/publications/en/uviguide.pdf

JS Beads, www.jsbeads.com

Locks of Love, www.locksoflove.org

Mary Quant, www.maryquant.co.uk

NPD Group, www.npd.com

Scott-Vincent Borba, www.borba.com

She-conomy, http://she-conomy.com

Society of Chiropodists and Podiatrists, www.feetforlife.org

Sonja de Lennart, http://sonjadelennart.com

Spanx, www.spanx.com

The New York Times, www.nytimes.com

Time, www.time.com

Timex, www.timex.com

Fairchild Dictionary of Fashion, third edition
By Charlotte Mankey Calasibetta and Phyllis G. Tortora